# the yoga healer

## REMEDIES FOR THE BODY, MIND, AND SPIRIT

FROM EASING BACK PAIN AND HEADACHES TO MANAGING
ANXIETY AND FINDING JOY AND PEACE WITHIN

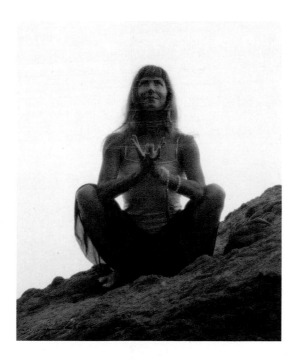

## Christine Burke

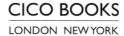

CICO BOOKS
LONDON NEW YORK

Published in 2017 by CICO Books
An imprint of Ryland Peters & Small Ltd
20–21 Jockey's Fields        341 E 116th St
London WC1R 4BW          New York, NY 10029
www.rylandpeters.com

10 9 8 7 6 5 4 3 2 1

Text © Christine Burke 2017
Design, illustration, and photography © CICO Books 2017

A CIP catalog record for this book is available from the
Library of Congress and the British Library.

ISBN: 978-1-78249-375-4

Printed in China

Editor: Marion Paull
Designer: Geoff Borin
Photographer: Erika Flores

Commissioning editor: Kristine Pidkameny
Senior editor: Carmel Edmonds
In-house design assistant: Kerry Lewis
Art director: Sally Powell
Production manager: Gordana Simakovic
Publishing manager: Penny Craig
Publisher: Cindy Richards

**Important health note**
Please be aware that the information contained in
this book and the opinions of the author are not a
substitute for medical attention from a qualified health
professional. If you are suffering from any medical
complaint or are worried about any aspect of your health,
or if you are pregnant, please ask your doctor's advice
before proceeding. The publisher and author can take
no responsibility for any injury or illness resulting from
the advice given or the postures demonstrated within
this volume.

# Contents

# the **yoga healer**

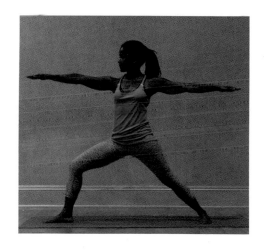

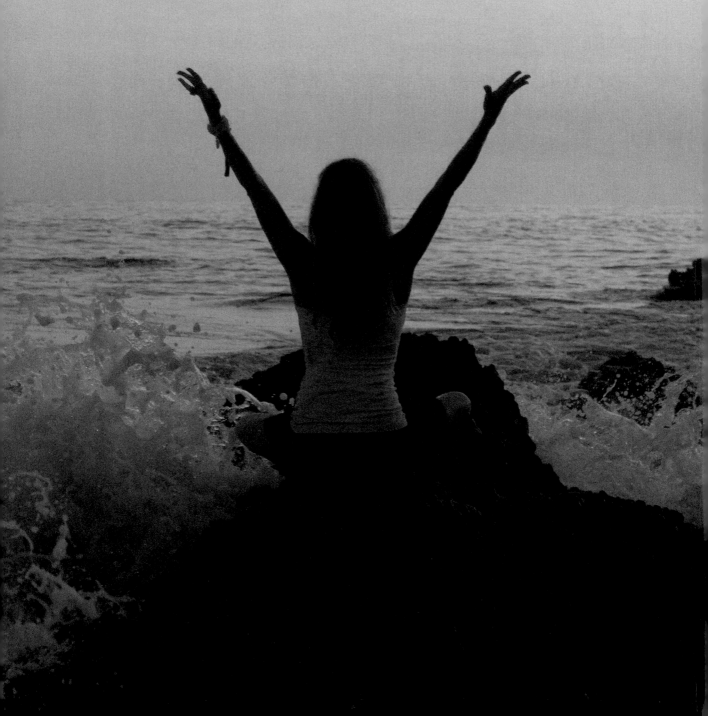

This book is dedicated to my family and my family of
students, who have inspired and encouraged me always;
And to my mother for her embodiment of courage and love,
to my father for challenging me to find a deeper strength,
to my husband for his wisdom, kindness and patience;
And to my Clementine—my angel, my guru.

# Introduction

Yoga is OLD—very old, roughly 6,000 years old—yet it is gaining popularity faster than you can say *Namaste*. This is because the themes and the practice of yoga are universal and timeless. Despite all the changes that have taken place over the centuries, whether magnificent or frightening, humanity has remained fundamentally the same. We long for connection and love, health and prosperity, peace and joy.

Yoga has a long list of benefits both physical and psychological. A yoga practice can improve posture, strengthen muscles, increase flexibility, lower blood pressure, decrease the likelihood of injury, improve lung capacity, relieve anxiety, lower stress levels, increase energy levels, and enhance mental clarity. The list goes on! Although the physical poses of yoga have gained the most attention in the West, they are but a rung on the ladder that leads to the ultimate and original goal of yoga, which is *moksha* or liberation. The definition of liberation is subject to many interpretations. For the purposes of this book, please consider what liberation means to you at this moment, and how it would positively affect your life to feel liberated.

We all have difficult moments, experience stress and loss, suffer temporary or chronic physical pain, and struggle with less than graceful moods at times. Wouldn't it be wonderful to carry around a tool belt filled with everything you need to address the various conditions that arise in your body, mind, and spirit in the course of a regular day? And wouldn't it be terrific if the remedy didn't come with a list of side effects and wasn't costly or time-consuming? And wouldn't it be really

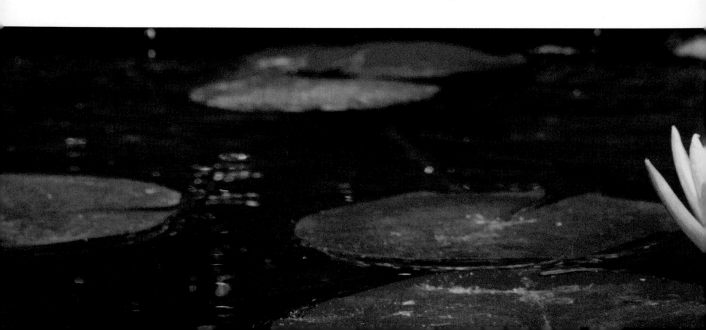

fantastic if you could turn this day around in 15 minutes or less? If you say "yes," this is where this book enters your life and makes it better. It is your companion and your guide.

Imagine that you could stop the momentum that has landed you with an aching back or stress headache, or has left you feeling disheartened and disappointed. Imagine that you could take your healing into your own hands right here and now. You can recover your equilibrium and start your energy moving toward wellness in a few moments. You can allow yourself to acknowledge your feelings and not become overwhelmed by them, creating more discord and conflict. This is the beauty of yoga. You can literally practice a breathing technique or short series of poses and get moving in the direction of feeling better right away—and I will show you how in this book.

Hatha yoga is often defined as an art and a science. The science is that we practice certain poses (asanas), breath practices (pranayama), and the quietening of the chatter of the mind

(meditation) in a way that produces proven benefits. The art is our personal expression, the way we use the tools that yoga provides. Many painters use a brush and yet no two paintings are identical.

The yoga in this book is hatha yoga as I practice and teach it. It is a simmering stew of all things yoga, based in tradition, and prepared for you with experience, love, humor, and passion. I have been blessed to share yoga with thousands of students and I have been fortunate to witness transformation and evolution every day. Feel free to pick up this book and flip to the condition that ails you or calls to you. You may also enjoy reading it all the way through. Whether you are a newcomer to yoga or a seasoned yogi, my prayer is that you will become more deeply acquainted with the healer in you, and that this relationship will infuse your life with wellbeing and many days of being well.

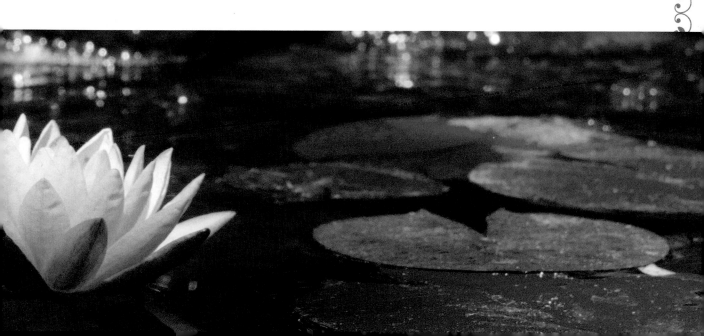

# How to Use This Book

A regular practice of yoga can be a life-changing and life-enhancing experience. While a traditional practice of one- or two-hour sessions is certainly something to consider and incorporate into your schedule if you can, there is much to be gained from brevity and consistency as well. Never underestimate how the power of a few focused minutes can transform your health and your outlook.

## Getting the best out of the book

This book can be used for on-the-spot remedies by simply flipping to the desired section and following the practice.

You can expand any of the practice remedies by adding a warm-up sequence (pages 16–22). This is particularly important if the remedy provided includes deeper or stronger poses, and I have noted where this is the case .

Use the cool-down sequence (pages 23–25) after the remedial poses for further relief of muscle tension and deep relaxation, or to prepare for a good night's sleep.

The key poses section (pages 9–13) describes foundational poses that will come up frequently in the book. It's a good idea to familiarize yourself with these poses.

Explanations of key concepts and practices are provided here (pages 14–15) so that you may better understand why these are included and how they are beneficial.

I have provided the English and Sanskrit names for poses where they first appear, and then the majority are referred to by their English name. There are a few exceptions, where the Sanskrit name is used more regularly in yoga classes, so I have used the Sanskrit throughout for those.

## Getting started with yoga

One of the best things about yoga is that it can be practiced anywhere and in any way. That being said, some things that will make it easier and more comfortable are a yoga mat, a yoga blanket and/or bolster, two yoga blocks, and a yoga strap. Wear comfortable clothing, without zippers or buttons, that you would normally wear to exercise in. Feel free to get creative, and never let a lack of props stand in your way of practicing yoga. If you can breathe, you can practice. You can find what you need online or in your local yoga studio. Some health food stores often sell yoga equipment, too.

# Key Poses

These poses come up again and again—
you will soon know them all!

### *Dandasana* (Staff Pose)

Sit with your legs together straight out in front
of you, and with your feet flexed (toes pointing
to the sky). Sit toward the front of your sitting
bones so that you don't slump into your lower
back. Place your hands alongside your hips on
the floor. Your arms may be bent or straight
with your palms or fingertips on the floor.
Keep your spine straight and press your legs
down toward the ground (**above right**). If you
feel lower back strain, you may find it more
comfortable sitting on a folded blanket (**right**).

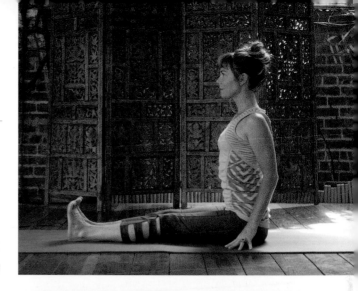

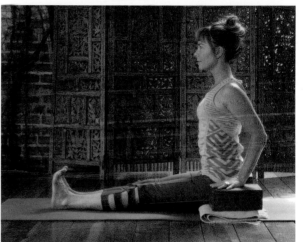

### Focus/Gazing Point (*Drishti*)

Set your eyes on one point in order to improve
concentration and balance, and cultivate peace
of mind.

### *Tadasana* (Mountain Pose)

Stand up tall with your feet together and your
arms extending energetically by your sides.
Balance on each foot equally from the inner to
the outer, from the ball to the heel. Firm your
legs. Set a focus point (*Drishti*) in the near
distance in front of you at eye height. Keep the
chest open, the shoulders back and down.

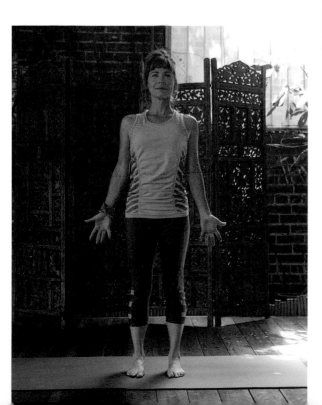

### *Sukhasana/Siddhasana* (Easy Pose and Accomplished Pose)

These variations are mainly used for meditation and breath work.

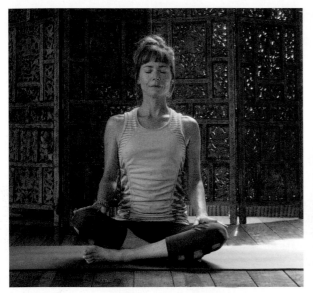

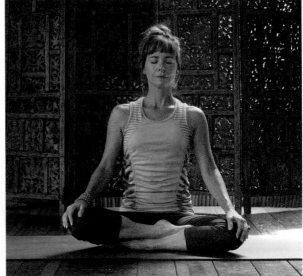

For *Sukhasana* (Easy Pose), sit with your legs straight out in front of you in *Dandasana*. Bend one leg and bring it in. Bend the other leg and cross it over the first one. Your legs should be crossed at the shins, and when you look down you should see a triangle between your legs. Keep a comfortable gap between your feet and your pelvis. You may wish to sit up on a folded blanket to avoid compression in the lower back, or tuck a blanket under your knees for more support.

For *Siddhasana* (which is a bit more advanced), begin in the same way as for *Sukhasana*, but when you bend your first leg, bring in the foot so that it lies snug to the opposite thigh. When you bend the other leg, the foot tucks in between the opposite calf and thigh. It's as if you are hiding your feet.

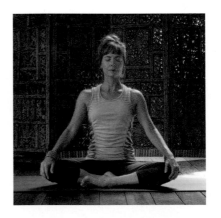

Another option that you will see in the book is a loose *Siddhasana*, where the legs are open wider than in *Sukhasana* and the feet are not tucked in but on the floor in front of you with the heels lining up.

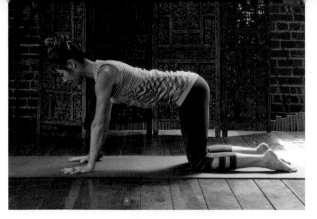

## Tabletop Pose (*Bitilasana*—Cow Pose)

This is simply coming to all fours, placing hands under shoulders with fingers spread wide and knees under hips with the tops of the feet on the floor. Although the closest translation in Sanskrit is Cow Pose, in this version the back is flat, not arched (see page 40).

## Standing Forward Fold (*Uttanasana*)

Stand in *Tadasana* with your feet either together or hip-width apart, and place your hands on your hips. Breathe in and as you exhale fold forward toward the floor, bending at the hips and aligning them over your ankles. Release your hands and clasp your elbows or place the hands on the floor near the outer edges of your feet. Keep your legs engaged and the shoulder blades pressed firmly into your back and moving away from your ears.

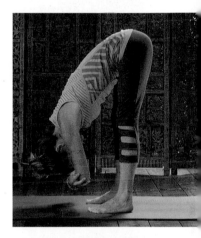

## Downward Dog (*Adho Mukha Svanasana*)

Begin on hands and knees in tabletop position with your hands directly under your shoulders, fingers spread wide like starfish, and your knees placed directly under your hips. Soften the space between your shoulder blades (think of a hammock) and engage your belly button. Without moving your hands, squeeze the arms toward each other and you will feel your biceps and triceps wake up. On an inhale, raise your hips and begin to straighten your legs. Push your chest toward your thighs and your heels toward the floor. Rotate your inner elbows to face toward each other. If you have very flexible or even double-jointed elbow joints,

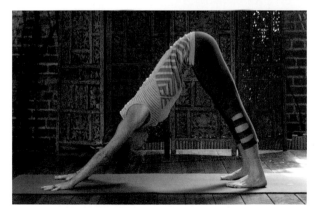

bend your elbows out slightly until the arms appear straight to the eye. This will engage the arms and protect the joints.

## Child's Pose (*Adho Mukha Virasana/ Balasana*)

For *Adho Mukha Virasana* (**right, top**), start on hands and knees and bring your big toes together, shifting your knees apart so that they are wider than your hips. On an exhale, draw your navel toward your spine, creating a dome in your back, as you ease your hips onto your heels. This creates more space in the lower back. Once you are settled, allow your back to flatten out naturally as you nestle into the pose. Your forehead is on the floor with your chin tucked in and the back of the neck long. You can leave your arms stretched out in front of you, hands flat on the floor and fingers spread wide like starfish, or lay them alongside your legs with your hands near your heels, palms up.

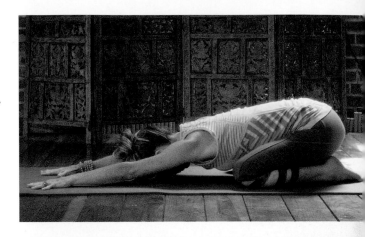

If your hips are high or you have trouble reaching the floor with your head, use a support, such as a folded blanket or block, under your forehead. If this pose is uncomfortable for your knees, you can use a bolster or folded blanket as a support: pull it into your pelvis and lay your torso along the support with your head turned to one side; your arms can be alongside your body with the palms facing up, or bring them forward, bend the elbows and "hug" the bolster (page 112). If your knees are still uncomfortable, roll up a blanket, towel, or article of clothing and place it snugly behind both knees before lowering your hips.

For *Balasana* (**right, bottom**), begin on hands and knees, but keep your legs together as you draw the navel to the spine and ease your hips

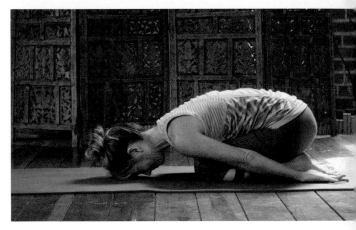

onto your feet. As with *Adho Mukha Virasana*, you can leave the arms outstretched or lay them alongside your legs, palms facing up.

### Hugging Knees to Chest (*Apanasana*)

Lie on your back and draw your knees in toward your chest. Wrap your arms around your legs and hug them as close as is comfortable for your knees. Keep your shoulder blades and head on the floor.

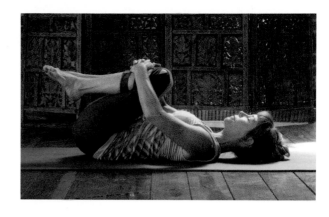

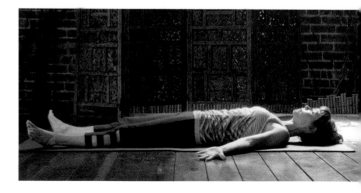

### Supine Twist (*Supta Matsyendrasana*)

Lie on your back with your knees drawn into your chest. Keep your left hand on your right knee and stretch your right arm out to the right at shoulder height. Shift your hips slightly to the right and, as you exhale, draw your right knee across your body to the left. Turn your head to the right. Keep your shoulder blades in contact with the floor and your chest open and facing upward. Repeat on the other side. This pose translates as Reclining Lord of the Fishes.

### *Savasana* (Corpse Pose)

Lie on your back with your head in line with your spine. Spread your legs apart, a little wider than your hips, with your feet rolling slightly open in a natural position. Extend your arms away from your body (about 8 inches/ 20 centimeters) with the palms facing up. Close your eyes and breathe naturally. Relax.

# Key Concepts and Practices

***Sthira Sukham Asanam*—Steady, stable, happiness, ease in the posture**

From the *Yoga Sutras* of Patanjali

When learning a breathing technique, a mudra, or the bandhas, it is like learning a pose—lean in with compassion, patience, and curiosity. Take your time, relax, and let it unfold for you over time. It is not something to be conquered but something to be experienced.

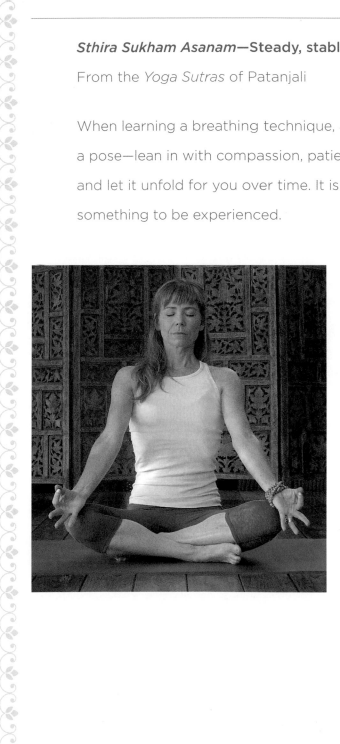

## PRANAYAMA

*Prana*: life force

*Yama*: restrain or control

This is the practice of controlling the breath through various techniques toward a particular goal, such as relaxation or energizing or balancing the body, mind, and spirit. *Prana* is translated as life force, vitality, and essence. It can be thought of as that which animates our being, and the breath is the way we finesse and fine-tune our life force. There are many more pranayama techniques than those offered in this book, but these are the ones I come back to time and again in my teaching and personal practice, and I find them to be essential.

## MUDRA

*Mud*: pleasure or delight

*Dra*: bring forth

The whole word means to seal in a gesture or attitude, so when practicing a mudra we are sealing in an attitude or gesture with pleasure and delight!

This term refers to the position taken with the hands and fingers toward a particular goal. The mudras work on a couple of levels. The position of the fingers and their relationship to one another stimulates the nerve endings and energy channels (the *nadis*) in the body. This can have an effect similar to reflexology, acupuncture, and pranayama in that it moves the life force (*prana*) through the body in a certain way. Another aspect is the intention set behind the mudras. By announcing to ourselves that we are holding, or sealing in, a particular focus, we have ingested that intention and brought clarity and energy to our desire. Mudras have been prevalent in many cultures for thousands of years, and we even use them unconsciously in our daily lives as we speak and our fingers tell the story of our feelings.

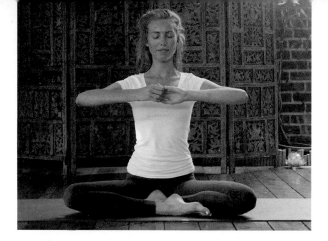

There is also a smaller collection of mudras for the body, of which a couple are described in this book. Body mudras are for sealing in a particular energetic intention by holding a physical position, which includes the whole body, not just the fingers.

## BANDHAS

This is the term for body locks, and the definition is to lock, hold, or tighten. You can think of it in terms of locking in the purity, goodness, light, and healing that the body is undergoing, and preserving this pure energy so that it doesn't easily dissipate or leak out. The bandhas enhance the yoga practice in many ways and are credited with producing many benefits. They help the practitioner to cultivate focus, heighten awareness, bring lightness and balance to the postures, tone and regulate the internal systems, and regulate the metabolism. They also help detoxification and digestion, among other things. The three major bandhas are root lock (*Mula Bandha*—pulling up the pelvic floor), the diaphragm ("flying up lock"/ *Uddiyana Bandha*), and throat lock (*Jalandhara Bandha*). The application of all three at once is Great Lock (*Maha Bandha*).

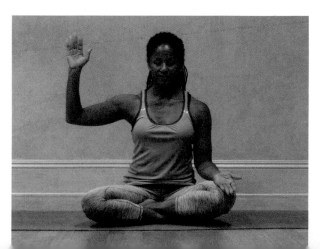

# Warm-up Sequences

Here are three sequences that you can use to warm up before any of the remedies in the book. The least strenuous is the Sun Salutations B variation; Classical Sun Salutations is intermediate level; and Sun Salutations A is the most strenuous.

## SUN SALUTATIONS B VARIATION
(*Surya Namaskar B variation*)

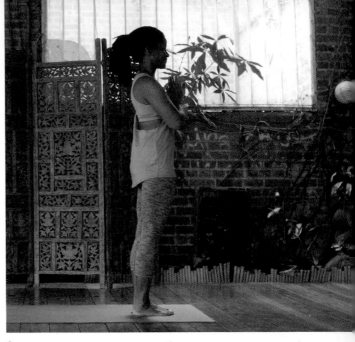

**1** Stand in *Tadasana* (page 9) with your feet together or hip-width apart, and bring your hands together in prayer position over your heart center (*Anjali Mudra*).

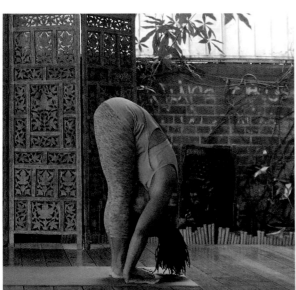

**4** Exhale and fold forward again into a Standing Forward Fold.

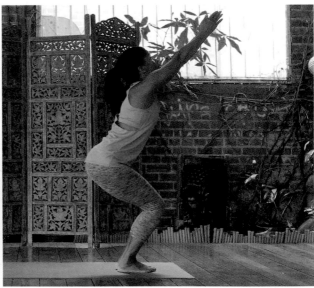

**5** Inhale to lift up your arms and bend at the hips, knees, and ankles, lowering your rear while stretching the torso upward. Exhale. Keep your arms active and in line with your ears—don't let them drift forward. This is the Chair or the Powerful Pose. Hold for 1–3 breaths.

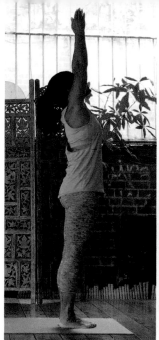
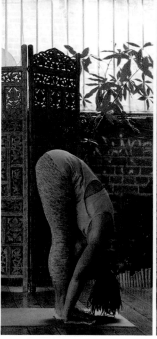
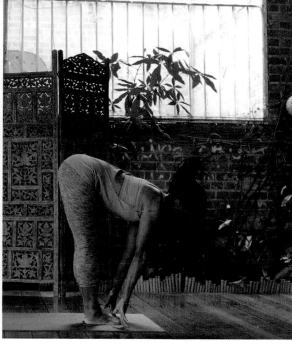

**2** On an inhale, sweep the arms out to the sides and overhead. As you exhale, bend forward from the hips into Standing Forward Fold (page 11). Bend your knees if your back is tender.

**3** Inhale and lift up your chest, lengthening your spine. Your arms are straight, and your hands are touching either the floor or your shins. This is a Standing Half Forward Fold.

**6** On your next inhale, lift straight up to standing, pushing firmly into your feet, arms stretching to the sky. Exhale as you bring your hands back to prayer position over your heart center (*Anjali Mudra*). Let your breath guide you into a rhythm and repeat as many times as you like with a minimum of 5 cycles.

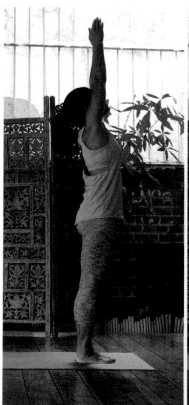
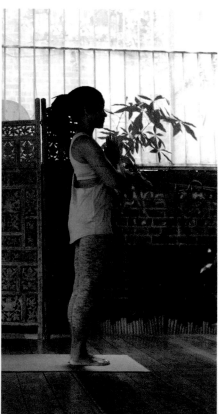

# SUN SALUTATIONS A (*Surya Namaskar A*)

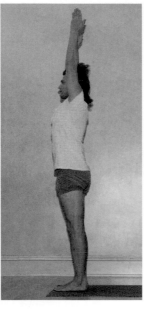
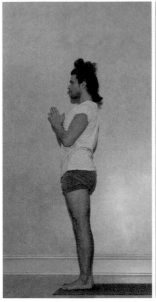
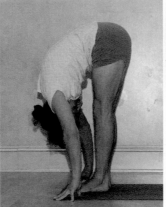
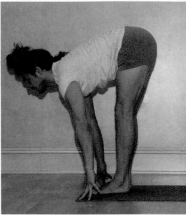

**1** Stand in *Tadasana* (page 9) with hands pressed together in prayer position over the heart center (*Anjali Mudra*). Inhale and sweep the arms out to the sides and overhead.

**2** Exhale and bend from the hips into a Standing Forward Fold (page 11).

**3** Inhale and lift your chest up, lengthening your spine. Your arms are straight, and your hands are touching either the floor or your shins. This is a Standing Half Forward Fold.

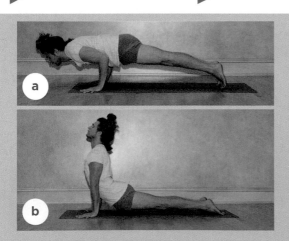
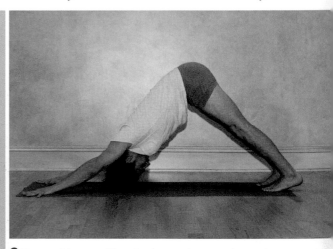

**4 and 5 alternative:** Jump from Standing Half Forward Fold to Low Plank as you exhale, stopping a few inches from the floor, elbows bent and triceps parallel to the floor (**a**). Press strongly into the floor and inhale as you pull your chest forward, straightening your arms and raising your legs off the ground. Just your hands and the tops of your feet are in contact with the floor. This is Upward Facing Dog (pages 150–51) (**b**).

**6** From either position, tuck your toes under and exhale into Downward Dog (page 11)—lift your hips and push your chest toward your thighs and your heels toward the floor, keeping your core strong. Take 1–3 breaths.

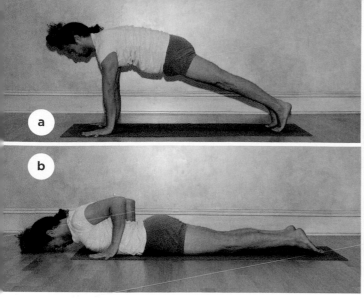

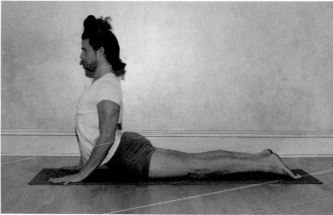

**4** Hold your breath and step back to High Plank (pages 101–102) (**a**). Your hands should be under your elbows, arms vertical, and the balls of your feet should be under your heels, legs straight. Your body should slope in a straight line from head to heels. Exhale as you lower to the floor, engaging your abdominal muscles and keeping your elbows in (**b**).

**5** From the floor, make sure your legs are active, toenails on the floor, root through your hips and pelvis, and inhale as you lift into Cobra Pose (pages 43–44).

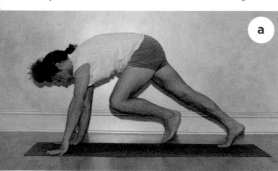

**7** On an exhale, either step or hop forward to your hands (**a**). Inhale as you stretch into Standing Half Forward Fold (**b**), exhale, and fold into Standing Forward Fold (**c**).

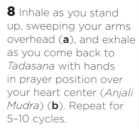

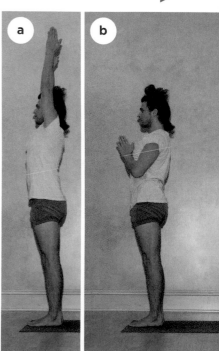

**8** Inhale as you stand up, sweeping your arms overhead (**a**), and exhale as you come back to *Tadasana* with hands in prayer position over your heart center (*Anjali Mudra*) (**b**). Repeat for 5–10 cycles.

# CLASSICAL SUN SALUTATIONS (*Surya Namaskar C*)

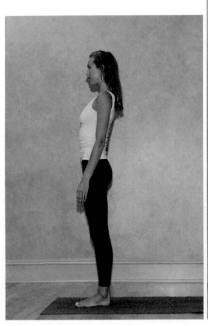

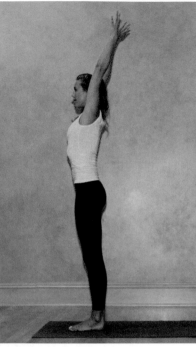

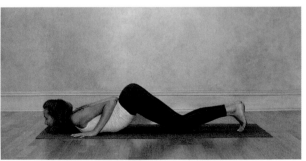

**1** Stand in *Tadasana* (page 9). Press hands together in prayer position over the heart center (*Anjali Mudra*), inhale, and either sweep the arms out to the sides and overhead or hook the thumbs and as you inhale dive the hands down and then up, arching your back a little if it feels safe to do so. Keep the legs strong and the core engaged.

**2** Exhale and fold from the hips into a Standing Forward Fold (page 11), bending the knees if the back is sensitive.

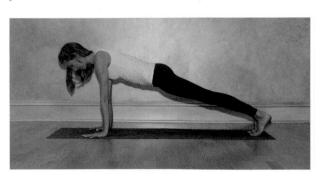

**6** Exhale and step back to High Plank (pages 101–102). Your wrists should be under your elbows, hands pointing forward, arms vertical, and the balls of your feet should be under your heels, legs straight. Your body should slope in a straight line from head to heels.

**7** Exhale as you lower your knees to the floor followed by your chest and chin.

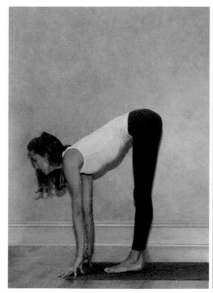

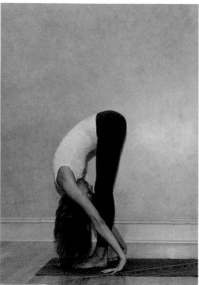

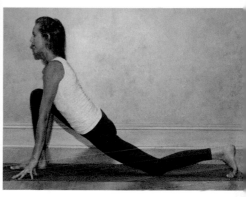

**3** Inhale and lift your chest up, lengthening your spine so that your back is flat. Your arms are straight, and your hands are on the floor or your shins. This is a Standing Half Forward Fold.

**4** Exhale and fold forward again into a Standing Forward Fold.

**5** Inhale and, bending the right leg, step the left leg back coming onto the knee. Keep the hands on the floor or sweep them overhead and slightly back.

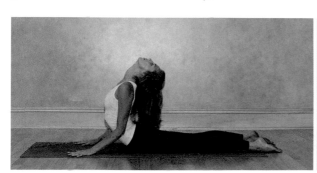

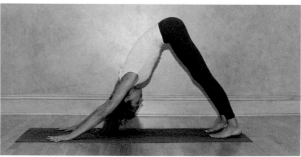

**8** Inhale as you slide your chest forward into Cobra Pose (pages 43–44) with your lower abdomen, pelvis and legs pressing into the floor. If it is comfortable, extend your neck and then release the head back. If not, look straight ahead.

**9** Exhale and push back to Downward Dog (page 11)— lift your hips and push your chest toward your thighs and your heels toward the floor, keeping your core strong.

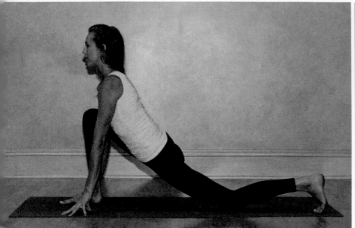
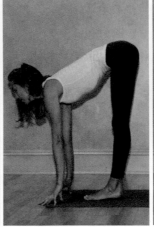
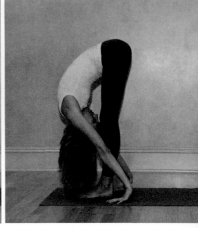

**10** Inhale as you bring the right leg forward between your hands. Either keep the hands there or lift them overhead. Exhale and return the hands to either side of your foot.

**11** Inhale as you step forward into Standing Half Forward Fold and exhale as you move into a full Standing Forward Fold (page 11).

**12** Either sweep the arms out to the sides or hook the thumbs in front of you and inhale as you sweep the arms up overhead. Bend the knees if your back is sensitive.

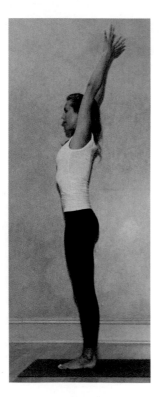

**13** Exhale as you bring the hands back to prayer position over heart center (*Anjali Mudra*) and finish in *Tadasana* (page 9). Repeat for 5–10 cycles, alternating which leg steps back to start.

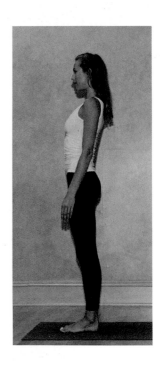

# Cool-down Sequence

This mini cool-down relaxes muscles and mind, which allows for an even deeper calm to settle in.

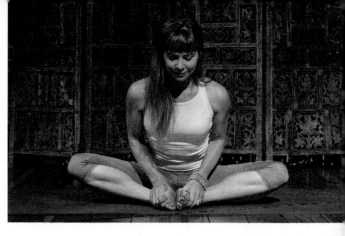

**1** Sit on the floor or a support and come into Butterfly Pose (*Baddha Konasana*, page 68) by bending your knees and bringing the soles of your feet together. Hold your feet and, for both of them, press your thumb into the depression under the ball of your foot between the big toe and second toe, which is roughly the middle. Aim for the most tender part. This acupressure point is good for calming an anxious mind and for general relaxation. As you press into your feet, extend your spine upward through the crown of your head. Then crease at your hips and stretch forward. Breathe 3–5 deep, slow breaths.

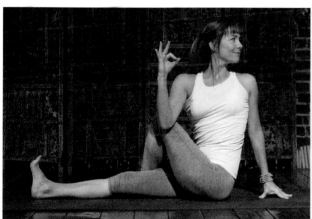

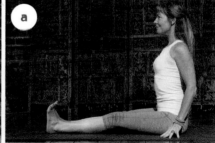

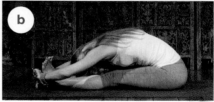

**2** Stretch your legs out in front of you for Half Lord of the Fishes (*Ardha Matsyendrasana*, page 64). If your lower back is strained or rounded, sit on a blanket or two. Bend your left knee and bring your left leg over your right, placing the foot on the floor outside of your right leg. Extend your right leg and press through the heel as you press your leg toward the floor. Support yourself by planting your left palm or fingertips on the floor (or a block) behind your back. Lift your right arm up to the sky, bend the elbow and hook it outside of your left knee. You can take *Jnana Mudra* here (for added focus) by connecting your thumb and index finger, or leave the fingers open. Sit tall and gaze over your left shoulder, or, if that is too much of a stretch for your neck, leave your chin over your chest. Take 3–5 breaths before you release and repeat on the other side.

**3** Now sit with both legs out in front of you in *Dandasana* (page 9) (**a**) and come to Intense Stretch of the West (*Paschimottanasana*, pages 64–65) (**b**). If you were using blankets for the last pose, stay on them here. Lengthen your spine and, as you inhale, extend your arms upward. On your exhale, crease at the hips and clasp your hands around your feet. If your back is sensitive or your hamstrings are tight, walk your hands in front of you alongside your legs until you feel a deep stretch without strain. Keep the legs active and the toes pointing up. Your head should remain in line with your spine. Take 3–5 breaths.

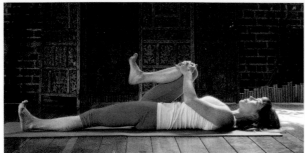

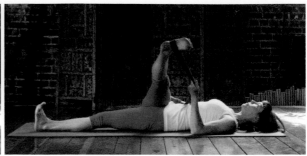

**4** Lie on your back for Reclining Hand to Big Toe Pose (*Supta Padangusthasana*, pages 52–53). Bend your right knee and draw it into your chest. Stretch your left leg out and flex your foot. Stay here for 1–3 breaths and then wrap the index and middle fingers of your right hand around your right big toe in yogi toelock (page 104) and stretch the leg up. If you cannot straighten your leg, use a strap, towel or T-shirt around the upper middle of your right foot. Hold the strap in each hand and slide the hands down enough for your chest to remain open and so that your shoulders are not tense. Hold this position for 5 breaths.

Then move the strap into your right hand, place your left hand on your left thigh to anchor it and let your right leg slowly release to the right. Keep both legs active as well as your core muscles and hold for 3–5 breaths.

Lift the right leg up, switch the strap to your left hand, and take your leg across the body (**above**). Hook your right thumb into your right hip crease and push away from your upper body to lengthen your side waist and deepen your stretch. Keep your lower back on the floor. Take 3–5 breaths.

Return to the center, hug the knee into your chest and repeat on the other side.

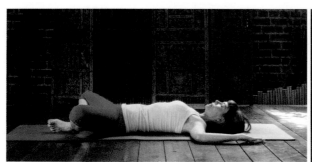

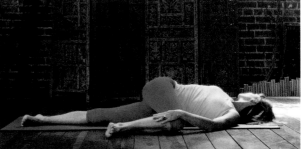

**7** Release your feet to the floor with the soles touching and the knees open for Reclining Butterfly (*Supta Baddha Konasana*). Stretch your arms out at shoulder height, or bend the elbows if you prefer. If you like, you can roll your head to one side for a few breaths and then the other.

**8** Draw your knees into your chest, extend your left leg out on the floor, and with your left hand draw your right knee across your body for Reclining Lord of the Fishes (page 13). Reach your right arm out at shoulder height and roll your head in that direction. Hold for 3–5 breaths, return to center, and repeat on the other side.

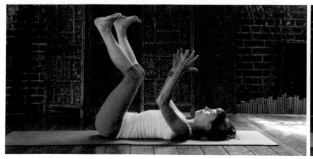 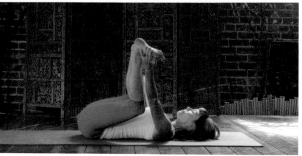

**5** Lie on your back, lift your arms and legs into the air with a bend in your knees and arms (ragdoll-style) and twirl your ankles and wrists. After a minute, reverse the direction of your twirl. This releases compression and tension in your joints and feels nice!

**6** From there, grab your feet or ankles, or even behind your knees for Happy Baby Pose (*Ananda Balasana*). Have your ankles right over your knees and your knees wide apart. Pull the legs toward the floor, keep the lower back in contact with the floor, and breathe 3–5 slow, happy breaths.

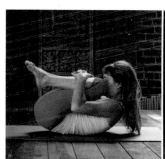 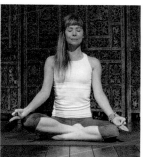

**9** Hug both knees into your chest and on an exhale, bring your forehead to your knees. Give an extra squeeze here and then release into *Savasana* (page 13) by stretching the body out evenly on the floor—arms about 8 inches (20 centimeters) from the body, inner thighs and feet gently rolling open, eyes closed.

**10** You may choose to finish in seated meditation. Let your breath be soft and natural and release all mental and physical effort. Surrender.

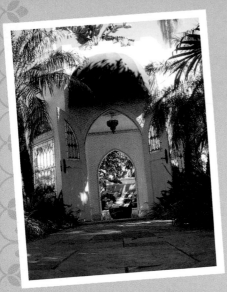

# PART 1

# Remedies for the Body

TOP TO BOTTOM

### Body

"The physical structure of a person or an animal, including the bones, flesh, and organs"

### Home

"The dwelling place or retreat of an animal"; "any place of residence or refuge: a heavenly home"

### Sacred

"Highly valued and important: deserving great respect"

As the tortoise carries his home on his back, we move through life inside of ourselves. Yogis say the body is a container for the spirit. In a place that resonates with light and love, a sacred space or spot in nature, the energy is palpable. You may wish to stay longer or even live there. In our most ideal circumstances, we would travel through life feeling comfortable and inspired in our bodies. Yet all too often we notice the body in a superficial way, or only when something has gone awry. Caretakers clean, water, nourish, and protect a sacred space so that the energy and light are clear and vibrant. When we attend to our physical health by caring for the body, we too shine with the vibrancy of that attention. In nature there is an organic and remarkable precision and art to the eco systems. Our bodies also have a blueprint for harmony and balance, and it is part of the yogic journey to gain the self-knowledge needed to recognize our inherent wellness and uncover our natural ability to heal ourselves.

To develop a healing relationship with our bodies is to acknowledge that we are divine (and miraculous) by nature, and this is the premise of the spirituality of yoga. We use the body, whatever its state, to find a deeper freedom. To honor and protect, to enjoy and appreciate, to embrace and find compassion for these magnificent temples allows us a portal to unity. Feel as though you are taking wedding vows? You may as well, for it is the one certain "till death us do part" relationship you will have. It's time to fall in love with your home.

In this section, we will use asanas (poses) along with mudras (hand gestures) and pranayama (breathing techniques) to relieve many common physical concerns. Come to your practice, however lengthy or brief, from a place of acceptance and curiosity whenever possible. Yoga is goal-oriented, but no goal is as accentuated as that of staying present with "what is." Whatever your hopes may be for alleviating the condition you find yourself in, remain open to the bounty of possibilities that may await you with your attention in the present moment. Breathe, be, and consider these words from the *Bhagavad Gita*, as spoken to the young warrior Arjuna:

*"Even these (obligatory) works should be performed without attachment to the fruits. This is my definite supreme advice, O Arjuna."*

# Headache

## THINK LESS, BREATHE MORE

Headaches may ambush us for a variety of reasons, but according to the Mayo Clinic, the grand prizewinner is (drumroll) stress! The good news is that we can lessen the impact of tension headaches, and often prevent them in the first place, through yoga. When we calm the body and mind, we soothe the highly charged nervous system, helping to restore harmony and peace of mind, which may decrease tension and pain.

### 1. Triumphant/Victorious Breath with Large Head Mudra (*Ujjayi Pranayama* with *Mahasirs Mudra*)

Sit comfortably cross-legged in *Sukhasana* or *Siddhasana* (page 10) or on a chair. Place your hands on your thighs, either palms up or palms down, depending on what feels most comfortable for you. Inhale through your nose as though your breath is entering your body through your throat. Do this by tuning your awareness to, and lightly constricting, your throat. Feel the sensation and listen for the sound of your own breath like a "whoosh" or ocean waves. Exhale in the same manner, listening for that sound. If you are having trouble hearing it, exhale through an open mouth as you would when fogging up your sunglasses to clean them. Then close your mouth and try again. Don't be concerned about getting it right. The most important thing is that you focus on your breath and relax.

After you have practiced a few rounds of *Ujjayi* breath, add the mudra. Touch your thumb, index, and middle fingers together. Fold your ring finger into your palm and extend your pinky finger. Do this on both hands and rest them on your thighs or knee facing up (**below**). Continue with *Ujjayi* breaths, pausing for a few

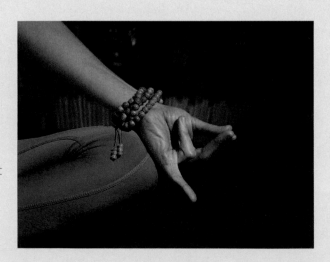

natural breaths in between, for 3–6 minutes. Hold the mudra for the entire time if possible. If you are experienced with *Ujjayi* breath, you can practice it for the entire 3–6 minutes and then rest.

**Modification:** If you prefer a simpler breath, place your hands on your belly and breathe deeply into the abdomen. Follow the rise and fall of your breath by feeling your hands move as you breathe.

## 2. Downward Dog (*Adho Mukha Svanasana*)

Nothing says yoga like Downward Dog. Here we are focusing on just one of its many benefits, as a remedy for headaches. Blood flows toward the upper extremities and the brain is refreshed as your head hangs and your neck stretches, while neck tension is released through gravity. This may produce tail wagging, which helps everything!

Follow the instructions on page 11. You may feel many sensations from restricted shoulders to zinging hamstrings—just keep breathing and allow the pose to ripen.

If you are struggling and straining, or feel tremendous pressure in your shoulders, you may want to try the modification below. If you are very flexible in the shoulders or back, make sure you don't overarch your back but keep your abdominal muscles strong, and don't let your shoulders drop toward the floor. Your arms should be strong and straight with no curves or bends.

Hold for 5–10 breaths; then bring the knees down and rest in Child's Pose (page 12). Repeat 3 times.

**Variation:** Especially useful as a remedy for a

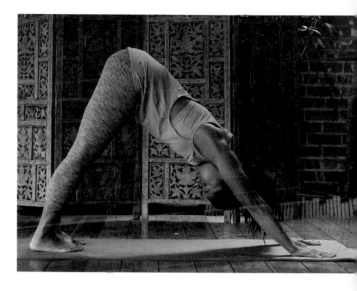

headache is to rest your head on some blocks or books in Downward Dog. Avoid causing strain by trying to reach the support with your head. It should feel easy to rest the head and still leave plenty of space around the shoulders.

**Modification:** If Downward Dog is too much for your shoulders or body for any reason, try using a wall for support (Wall Dog). Press the palms of your hands against the wall at shoulder height and shoulder-width apart. Step back—feet at hip-width, toes pointing forward—allowing your hands to slide down the wall, until your arms and trunk form a straight line, and your legs are perpendicular. Hold for 5–10 breaths and then rest. Repeat 1–3 times.

## 3. Legs up the Wall or Inverted Action (*Viparita Karani*)

This rejuvenating asana is my personal power nap. It is a tremendous immune-system booster and a wonderful neutralizer that can boost your energy or ground and calm you. Sometimes called "Inverted Lake Pose," referring to the area below the navel, the second, sacral chakra (*Svadhisthana*), it can produce the same sensation as focusing on a glassy, ripple-free lake, releasing tension in the body and mind. Try visualizing a beautiful, serene lake and imagine your breath as a gentle breeze that does not disturb the surface of the water.

Sit with your left hip against the wall. You can be on the floor (**below left**) or on a firm blanket or bolster (**below**). Put your weight onto your hands and arms as you swing your legs up the wall until you can lie back on the floor. Your lower back should be on the bolster or floor. If your hamstrings or back feel strained or you are having to make an effort to hold the pose, move yourself a few inches away from the wall and let your legs rest on an incline. You may also find it more comfortable to open the legs into a slight V shape. Hold for 5–10 minutes with your focus on the gentle rise and fall of your breath.

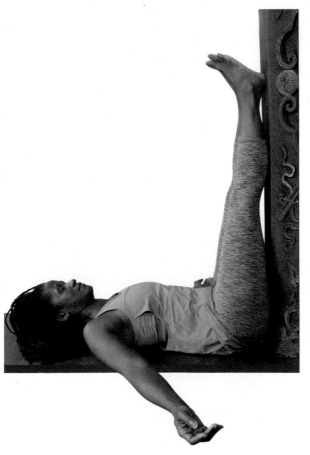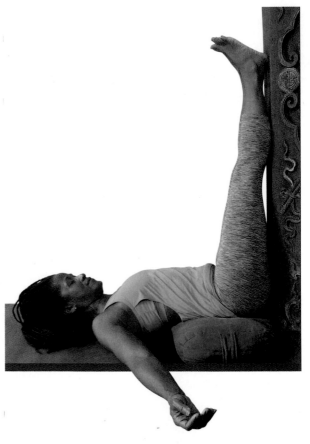

# A Pain in the Neck

## IS A PAIN IN THE NECK!

When you are suffering from a sore or stiff neck, it can be hard to ignore it and carry on with a stiff upper lip. After all, your neck supports your head and the ability to turn your head is pretty crucial, especially while driving. Whether you've slept yourself into a predicament, are suffering from a sudden spasm, or have chronic neck pain, try this sequence and maybe you can kick that pain in the neck in the asana!

### 1. *Sukhasana* with neck stretch and roll

Sit on the floor with legs crossed in *Sukhasana* (page 10). If it is more comfortable, sit on a blanket, block, bolster, or firm pillow. You may also wish to support your knees with blocks. Sit tall with a straight spine and soften your ribs into your body to avoid arching your back.

Rest your left hand on your left thigh or knee. Reach straight up with your right arm and bend the elbow to catch your left ear in the palm of your right hand. Ease your head toward your right shoulder. Don't yank your head or push down with your hand. Let gravity do the work of stretching the muscles on the left side of the neck while you focus on 5–10 breaths (**a**). Then slide your right palm to your right temple and carefully lift your head back to center. Repeat on the other side.

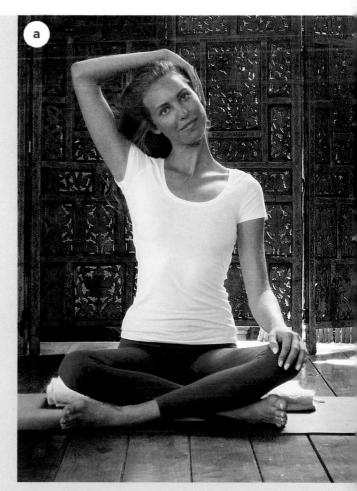

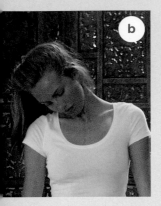 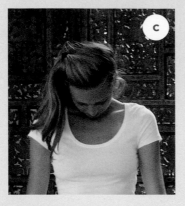 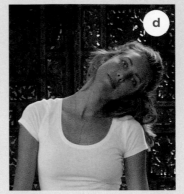 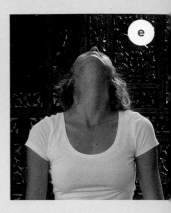

When you are finished with the pose, do three slow head rolls in one direction and then reverse for three more (**b, c, d, e**).

**Modification:** If this feels uncomfortable or you have a neck injury, do half head rolls from ear to shoulder along the chest and back rather than all the way around, which, for some, can be aggravating to the cervical vertebrae.

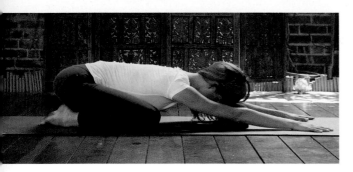

## 2. Child's Pose (*Adho Mukha Virasana*)

Ah, the wisdom of the child. This pose is always a wise choice to elevate your body and spirit. It can be done on the floor, with a few props or makeshift accessories if they make it better for you.

Follow the instructions on page 12 and stay in the pose for as long as you like.

**Variations:** For an elevated version, place your forehead on a block or stack of books so that your neck is in line with your spine and your chin is tucked slightly in toward your chest (**left**). For a superplush variation, a bolster or several blankets are required. Draw the support in between your knees up to your groin or abdomen and lean forward so that your torso and head are lying along the prop. Turn your head to one side for 1–2 minutes and then to the other side for 1–2 minutes (page 112).

**Modifications:** If you have any discomfort in your ankles, place a blanket beneath your feet. If your knees or quadriceps are tight, place a blanket or something similar evenly and snugly behind your knees before taking your hips back.

## 3. Bridge Pose (*Setu Bandhasana*) variation

Lying on your back, bend your knees so that your feet are directly under your knees and parallel to each other. Rest your arms by your sides and position your face toward the ceiling with the back of your neck long. Do not jut your chin upward. On an inhale, lift up your hips and take your right arm all the way back behind you so that the back of your hand touches the floor. At the same time, slowly roll your head to the left, away from your arm (**a**). On your exhale, bring your hips down and your arm back by your side as your head returns to center. Repeat on the other side to complete one cycle (**b**). Do 4–6 cycles.

Move slowly and synchronize your movements to your breath. Think of this as a dry-land backstroke and get into a rhythm as you would while swimming. This "vini style" sequence is wonderful for the neck and shoulders and soothing to the mind.

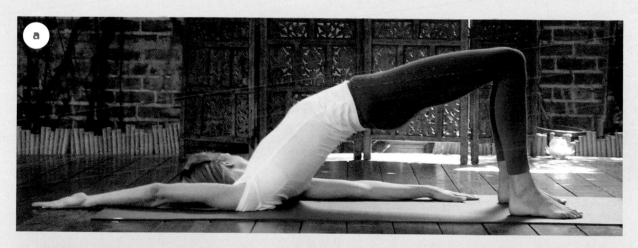

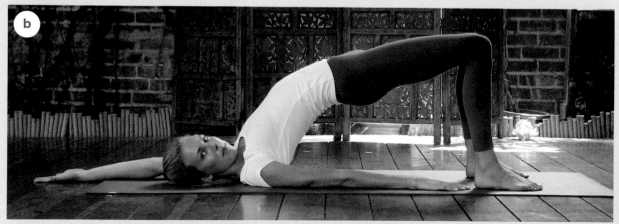

# Tight Throat

## FEEL FREE TO EXPRESS YOURSELF

The fifth chakra (energy center) in the throat, called *Vishuddha*, is our link to expressing ourselves. When the voice feels constricted or compromised, or we lose it, feelings of frustration, isolation, and even depression may soon follow. Your voice can be affected by stress, weight gain, age, diet, medications, environmental factors, and allergies. However, as we know, yoga lowers stress levels and promotes relaxation, and these beneficial effects may be felt in the throat just like anywhere else. Also, like any muscle group, the vocal cords can weaken without proper exercise. So, beside resting, warm tea, and honey, try this sequence of exercises.

### 1. Bee Breath (*Brahmari* Breath)

This pranayama is wonderful for relieving stress and sends a healing vibration through the vocal cords and chest. It can be practiced seated, on a chair or the floor, or lying down. Close your eyes, or keep them open but relaxed if you prefer. Place one hand on your heart and one hand on your belly. Inhale, and as you exhale make a deep humming sound like a bee. Hum from the chest and belly more than from the lips. Let the "breath buzz" fade out naturally. Do not strain for the sound to last, rather let it softly and naturally fade in the way a buzz from a bee fades as it flies farther away from you. Do 3–5 rounds. Then spend a few moments listening to your inner self and see what may arise for you.

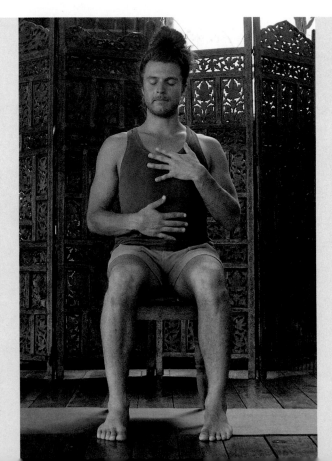

## 2. Shoulder Stand (*Salamba Sarvangasana*)

Known as the "Queen of the Asanas," shoulder stand has many lofty attributes and benefits associated with regular practice. If you are experiencing chronic throat troubles, work toward a regular practice of 3–4 times per week or more.

Place one or two folded blankets in the middle of your mat. If you like, fold your mat back over the blankets, leaving a few inches of blanket showing at the top (as on page 173). This will help your shoulders stick to the mat and stay aligned. Lie with your head off the blankets and your shoulders on them with a two-inch space between your shoulders and the top edge of the blanket. Sweep your legs over your head so your toes touch the floor, supporting your low to mid-back with your hands. This is Plow Pose (*Halasana*) (**a**). Draw your elbows in line with your shoulders as much as your shoulders will allow without strain. Distribute the weight between your arms and the back of the head and raise your legs, reaching up through the balls of the feet (**b**). Your arms, core, and legs should be active but not straining. Endeavor to bring your legs high enough to get your chest near your chin, which brings a balancing effect to the thyroid and aids circulation to the throat. Relax your face and listen to your breath for 5–10 breaths, working up to 3 minutes eventually.

**Variation:** For anyone who has neck, wrist, or shoulder injuries, it may be preferable to use a block—try it anyway, just because it combines a backbend with shoulder stand and is delicious.

Begin by lying on your back, knees bent, feet close to your hips. Lift your hips, shoulders still on the floor, and bring a block underneath your sacrum (a neat rectangular area in your lower

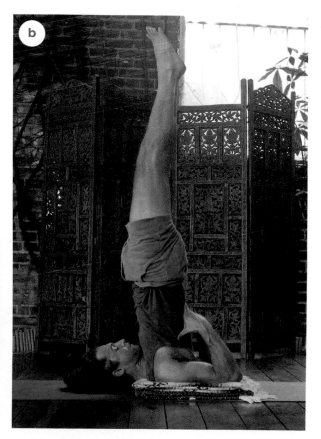

back designed perfectly for this!). You may need to explore to find the proper height and placement (not near your kidneys); then settle gently onto the block. Keep your chest lifted and your coccyx lowered. Lift your legs up so that they are directly in line with your hips, feet flexed and arms by your sides (page 61, **d**). Keep a firm pressure on the block with your sacrum and the chest lifted to avoid the block digging into your back. This should feel good and not be difficult to hold. If it is, replace it with Legs up the Wall (page 30).

### 3. Supported Fish (*Salamba Matsyasana*) with throat chakra meditation

Position a bolster, rolled-up blanket, or block where your shoulder blades will be when you lie on the floor. Then, from *Dandasana* (page 9)—sitting spine straight, legs straight out in front of you, feet flexed—lower yourself onto your set-up, and use your hands to press your thighs down and toward your feet. If you find your neck needs more support or your head needs some height, place another rolled-up blanket or towel behind your neck or under your head. Arms may be out to the side, bent at the elbows, palms up.

Once you are in the pose, close your eyes and take your attention to your throat chakra. If you are able and so inclined, try to visualize your favorite version of turquoise at your throat center—it could be a body of water or a gemstone, or just a free-floating color—and take a few breaths. If this is difficult for you, don't fret, just focus on the physical center of your throat. Then open your mouth and chant "ham" (pronounced "hum") so that the "mm" sound at the end is drawn out in the same way as chanting "om." Let the sound taper off as you did with the Bee Breath (page 34). "Ham" is the "seed sound" or *bija* mantra of the throat chakra. *Bija* mantras are used as healing tools on a cellular level, and they can activate and balance the energy centers in a healing way. Chant 5–8 times. If you prefer, do this lying flat on your back rather than in the pose.

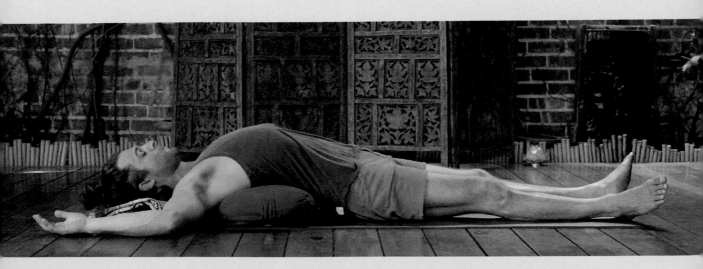

# Shoulder Tension

## CARRYING THE WEIGHT OF THE WORLD

Ever feel like you have too much on your shoulders? Or find yourself flinching in traffic? Responsibility has a way of settling into and onto the shoulders. Or maybe your love of weightlifting has rendered you able to lift small mountains but unable to scratch your back! Whatever the reason may be, the chronic shrug position can be painful and disrupt your happy flow. So let's get those shoulders rolling easily again and lighten your load!

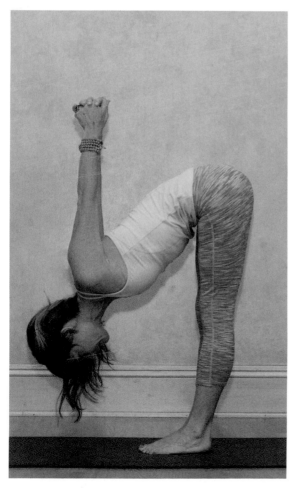

### 1. Standing Forward Fold (*Uttanasana*) with hands clasped

Stand tall in *Tadasana* (page 9) with your feet hip-width apart. Draw your navel in toward your spine. Clasp your hands behind your back. Inhale and on your exhale bend from the hips into a standing forward fold. If your back or hamstrings are tight, or you have been sitting awhile, bend your knees a little. Allow your breath to guide your shoulders to their optimum stretch away from your back. On an inhale lift your shoulders away from the floor, leaving space around your neck. Take 5 slow breaths and then release your arms to the floor and roll up slowly with bent knees.

**Modification:** For those with low back injury or extreme sensitivity, Wall Dog would be a better choice (page 29).

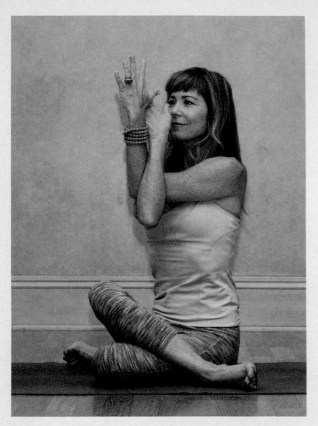

## 2. Eagle Arms (*Garudasana Arms*)

This pose can be done standing or seated. The standing version is done in *Tadasana* (page 9). For the seated version, come to hands and knees and place your left knee behind your right, sitting back between your feet with the right knee stacked on top of the left. Place your feet in line with each other on either side of your hips.

Whether standing or seated, as you inhale, stretch your arms wide at shoulder height with your palms facing up. Hold there with the arms outstretched for 3 breaths. Concentrate on rotating the inner arms up toward the sky and keeping the palms wide and facing directly up.

Then, on an exhale, wrap your arms with the left arm over the right, bend your elbows, and face the back of the hands toward each other. Your elbows should be parallel to the floor and chest high. Move your left hand to the left and your right hand to the right until your right pinky passes your left thumb, and place the fingers of your right hand into the palm of your left as much as is possible for you. Take 5 deep breaths here, gazing directly in front of you, and then slowly release the pose. Let your arms hang by your sides and relax for a few moments before repeating on the other side (legs as well, in the seated version).

**Modification:** Follow the above instructions for Eagle Arms from the comfort of a firm chair— perfect for a quick refresher at work!

## 3. Pranic Shoulder Bath

This dynamic sequence brings mobility to the shoulders and is also therapeutic for the wrists and hands. It can be practiced standing and include a forward fold for a whole-body experience, or modified to a seated version.

If standing, begin in *Tadasana* (page 9) with hands in *Pushpaputa Mudra*—hands together, palms open. Otherwise, sit on your heels, toes uncurled. On an inhale, extend the mudra straight out in front of you to arm's length (**a**) and then lift your arms straight up overhead, maintaining the mudra (**b**). Holding your breath, slowly flip the wrists so the backs of the fingers touch and briefly point toward your head (**c**); then fully stretch the arms back up again with the backs of the hands pressed together as far as you are able (**d**). On an exhale, open your arms wide and bring them down by your sides in a wide circle (**e**, **f**). If standing, fold forward, hingeing at the hips. Then slightly bend your knees and roll up to *Tadasana*.

Maintain a solid connection between the movement and the breath, and practice as many as you like with a minimum of 3 rounds.

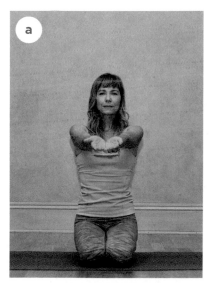

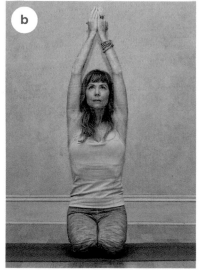

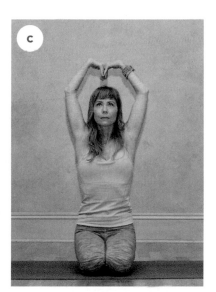

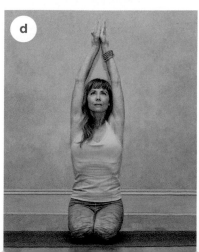

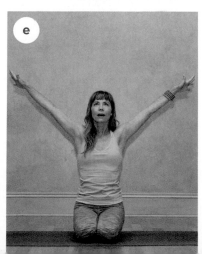

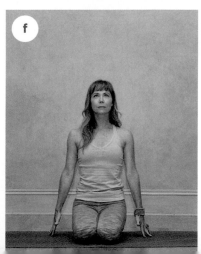

# Upper Back Pain
## POSTURE CHECK!

The upper back (thoracic spine) can morph into a block of ice seemingly overnight. It protects the vital organs in the chest by being a stable and less flexible point in the spine, but when our modern lives lead us to spend hours hunched over a desk or table, it's time to sit up (literally) and take notice. So the first order of business is to practice actually sitting up straight more often. This will tone your abdominal muscles, strengthen and support your spine, and make you feel better in general. After you have taken the posture check, move on to these asanas and melt into some relief.

### 1. Crooked or Churning Wheel, or Cat Cow (*Chakravakasana*)

Poses that address the spine seem so simple and yet are so beneficial. Such is the case with Cat Cow. Begin on all fours in the tabletop position with hands under shoulders and knees under hips. Relax your belly and soften the upper back while opening the chest and inhaling. Keep your shoulders back from your ears and tilt your head up slightly but not so much that you are crunching your cervical spine by collapsing your head onto your neck. Take care not to overarch your lower back, but rather concentrate on opening the chest and relaxing the abdomen. This is Cow Pose (**a**).

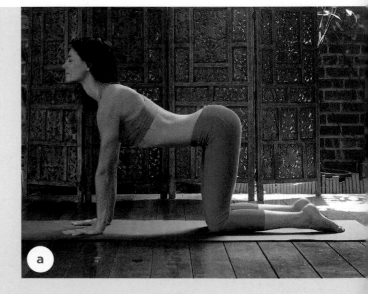

As you begin to exhale, move into Cat Pose (think scary Halloween cat) by tightening your abdominals and rounding your spine up toward the ceiling. Push into the earth with your hands, shins, and knees and let your head hang down (**b**). In both positions your arms stay straight. Practice 5–10 rounds, then rest in Child's Pose (page 12).

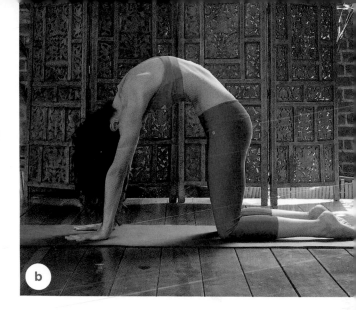

## 2. Extended Child's Pose (*Utthita Adho Mukha Virasana*) with arm variation

In addition to melting the thoracic spine, you will get a deep shoulder opener and neck release with this variation. Starting from hands and knees in the tabletop position, bring your big toes together and set your knees wide apart. Sit back on your heels, bend your elbows, placing them on the floor, forearms upright, and bring your palms together in *Anjali Mudra*, the prayer position, right over your elbows (**below**). Your forehead is on the floor.

Breathe deep, even breaths while you thaw the icy stiffness in your upper back. For some this will be a deep stretch, while for others it will render Child's Pose more comfortable.

**Modification:** For a deeper stretch, place your elbows on some blocks or books, keeping your forehead on the floor (**below right**).

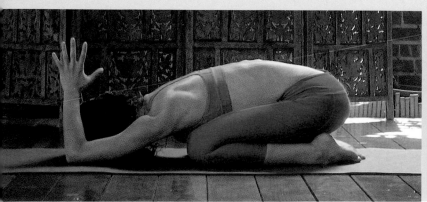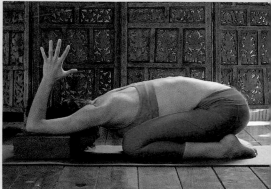

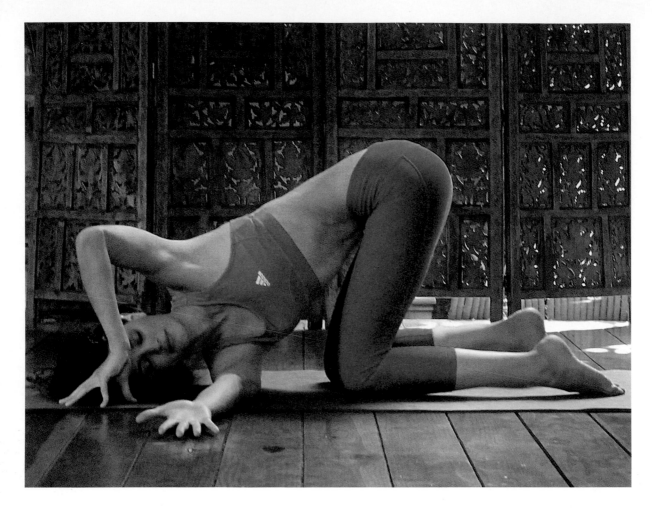

### 3. Revolved Child's Pose—Thread the Needle
### (*Parsva Balasana*)

Although this pose might be renamed "awkward asana," it is a wonderful upper back twist and stretch if you can relax into it. Beginning, as we so often do, on hands and knees, first lift your right arm out to the side and then bend it underneath your left arm. Make sure your left hand is directly beneath your left elbow with the fingers spread wide. Rest your right shoulder and the right side of your head comfortably on the floor, keeping the back of the neck long by slightly tucking your chin into your chest. Square your hips, which most likely means drawing your left hip back. Press your left hand into the floor to increase the twist without shifting your hips. Take 3–5 mindful breaths before unthreading and repeating on the other side.

# Tight Chest

## OPEN YOUR HEART

Another casualty of the unofficial pose I like to call "hunchasana" is the chest. When we collapse the chest from chronic slouching, the muscles in the chest wall get tight and this restricts the flow of blood and oxygen, leaving us a little deflated in body and spirit. The body also takes this shape when the mind is under duress and as a protective mechanism during times of sadness. Think of the position you are likely to take when crying—rarely do we stand up straight with an open chest to cry beyond the age of three! So a wonderful way to expand your physical heart center and boost your mood is to practice a heart opener or three.

### 1. Cobra Pose (*Bhujangasana*)

Lie flat on the floor with your forehead on the ground and your hands, pointing forward, right beneath your shoulders, elbows bent backward. Lengthen your legs behind you, extending directly out from your hips, and place all ten toenails on the floor (**a**). Rooting into your hips and pelvis, inhale as you rise up like a cobra slowly emerging to fan its chest (**b**).

Keep firm pressure into the floor from your pelvis to your feet, because this is the foundation from which you can open your chest. It is not necessary to straighten your

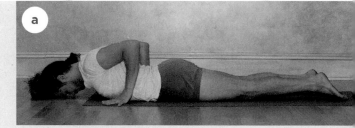

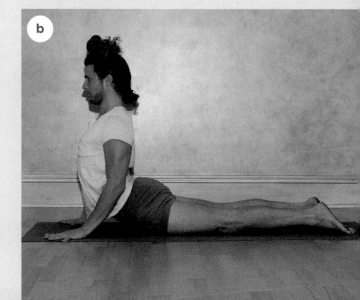

arms, and for some people not desirable because it can compromise the lower back. So your arms may be bent or straight, depending on how comfortable your low back feels. Seek to open your chest and strengthen your upper back muscles by focusing on the breath and staying tuned in to your sensations. Hold for 3–5 breaths, exhaling as you come down. Repeat 3 times. For a little extra pizzazz and to relax your jaw, you can make a hissing noise as you lower out of the pose.

## 2. Cow Face (*Gomukhasana*)

In its traditional form, this pose is practiced on the floor, but you can practice just the arm positions while sitting on a chair or standing. Choose what is most reasonable for you.

For the traditional version, come to the tabletop position on hands and knees and bring your knees together. Cross your left leg behind your right, making your knees snug. Move your hands out to the sides slightly and gently lower yourself back onto your sitting bones. Adjust your feet, keeping them flexed, heels toward hips, as much as possible. You may find it more comfortable for your hips to sit on a block, books, or a folded blanket.

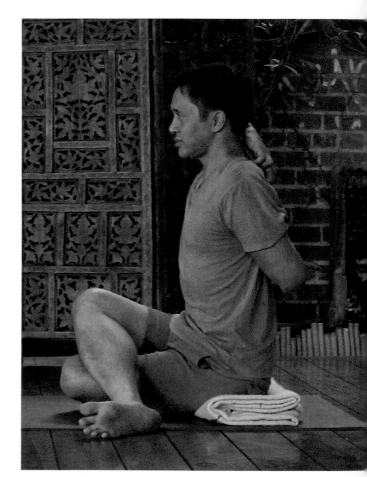

Stretch your arms straight up above your head. Bring your left arm down and bend it up behind you, palm facing out, as if you were trying to scratch your back. Bend your right arm directly down behind your back and clasp fingers. If you can't reach so that clasping eludes you, use a towel, yoga strap, or even your shirt to bridge the gap. Avoid puffing out the chest and therefore arching the back by softening the ribs into the body and keeping your belly button in. Bring your right arm as close to your head as possible and point the elbow up. Beside opening the chest, this is quite a rigorous shoulder opener, so move slowly and with the breath as you move into and out of the pose. Repeat on the other side, reversing the position of both the legs and the arms.

**Modification:** This crossed-knees version should not be practiced if you have an active knee injury. Sit on a chair, feet flat on the ground and parallel (**right**). If you have an injured shoulder, simply clasp the arms behind your middle back, holding the forearms.

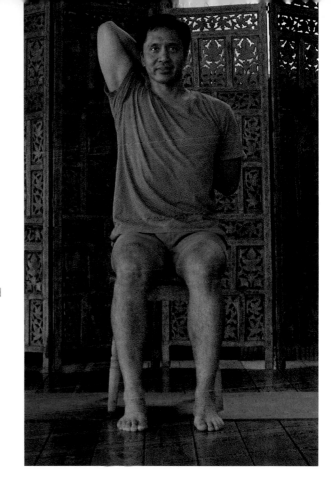

### 3. Supported Fish (*Salamba Matsyasana*)

This expansive and rejuvenating heart opener is one of my favorite poses of all time. Follow the instructions on page 36 to get into the pose. Once there, visualize the way a fish leaps out of the water and allow that freedom and lightness to come into your chest as you remain anchored through your legs. Enjoy your breath flowing through the lungs like gentle waves in the ocean. Stay in the pose for 1–3 minutes before easing onto one side, bending your knees, and rolling up to a seated position.

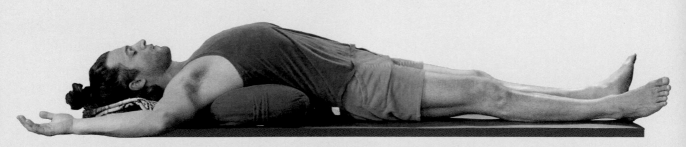

# Sore Hands, Wrists, and Fingers

LESS TEXT, MORE STRETCH!

This is an affliction of the age of technology! Maybe your fingers do most of your talking, or you suffer from arthritis, or play a sport where you engage in a repetitious activity that puts stress and strain on certain joints and tendons. Even yoga practiced improperly can be a culprit. Perhaps you have sustained an injury resulting in stiffness and joint pain or even carpal tunnel syndrome. Fortunately, there is a scenic road out of this tricky terrain! Maintaining flexibility and strength is key to keeping your fingers, hands, and wrists nimble and comfortable, so give your digits some TLC as often as you can.

## 1. Blooming Lotus Bud Mudra

Sit comfortably on a chair or with legs crossed and spine straight in *Sukhasana* or *Siddhasana* (page 10). Bend your arms so that the tips of your elbows land near your bottom ribs. Your forearms extend away from you, and your shoulders should be relaxed. Bring the tips of all five fingers of each hand together into Lotus Bud Mudra. Relax your eyes to closed, or almost closed if that is more comfortable for you. Press your fingertips firmly into each other as you inhale. Pause briefly at the top of your inhale, and as you exhale through your mouth, spread your fingers slowly so that your palm is completely outstretched. Begin your inhale from there, drawing your fingers closed again, and then repeat the exhale, opening your

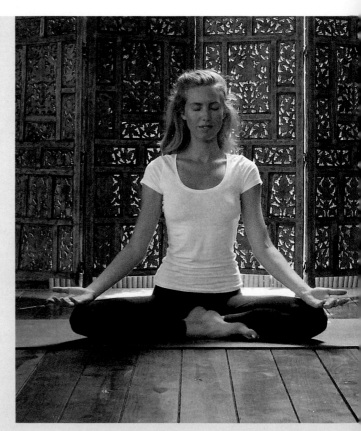

hands. Try holding the image of a blooming lotus flower in your mind's eye.

This meditation and breath practice is a way to invoke a feeling of awakening into the moment with new appreciation, and connects us to nature and the natural flow of life. By stimulating the nerve endings of the fingers during the bud part of the mudra, it encourages blood circulation in the hands and awakens fresh energy. When you spread the hands open, the tendons, muscles, and tissue of the hands, wrists, and fingers stretch. Repeat as many times as you like with a minimum of 5 cycles.

## 2. Half Sideways Hand Pose (*Ardha Parsva Hastasana*)

Stand straight in *Tadasana* (page 9), feet together or hip-width apart, your left side to a wall and at one arm's length from it. Place your left palm on the wall with your fingers pointing toward the ceiling and a small bend in your elbow. Keeping your palm as flat to the surface of the wall as you can and rolling your left shoulder blade down your back, begin slowly to straighten your arm (**a**). If your palm loses connection with the wall, bend your elbow until your palm is flat again. If it is easy to keep the palm flat, turn slightly away from the wall, still in *Tadasana* (**b**). Hold for 5–10 breaths and then go back to your original position.

Bend your elbow again and, if possible, turn your hand so that the fingers point behind you. Then slowly push the hand into the wall until the arm becomes straight or nearly straight (**c**). It will feel as if you are trying to push the wall away from you. Keep your shoulder blade down, your navel tucked in, and breathe! If you are able to, you can turn slightly away from the wall here, too. Take 5–10 breaths and then shake your arm out and repeat on the other side. If it is too intense to turn the hand back with the fingers pointing behind you, just hold longer with the fingers in the upward position.

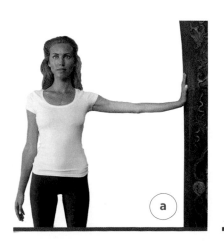

(a)

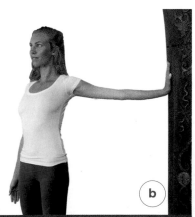

(b)

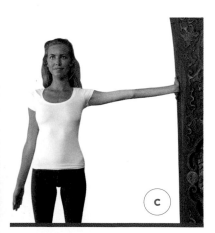

(c)

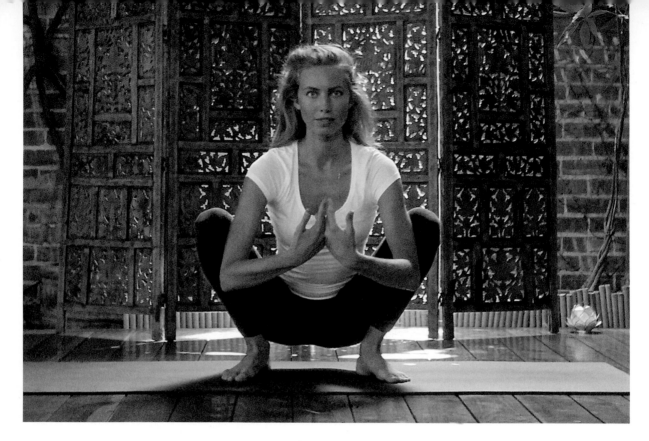

### 3. Garland Pose (*Malasana*) with Mudra for Inner Strength

This mudra is especially delightful practiced in Garland Pose for the added hip stretch and lower back release. However, if this is not feasible for you, it can be done seated or even lying down for a restful moment.

For Garland Pose, squat with your feet as close together as possible without causing strain to your knees. Your knees should be wider than your hips. If your heels don't touch the floor, place a rolled-up blanket, mat, article of clothing, or a block underneath your heels until you feel supported with some weight in the heels. Place your elbows inside your knees and press the backs of the hands into each other. Use your elbows to keep your hips open. If your thumbs touch in this mudra, that's fine, but do not force them to do so. Keep the hands active and the fingers stretched with your pinkies nestled into your sternum. Focus on the feeling of the breath in your chest. Your eyes can be closed or find a focus point (*drishti*) slightly above your eyeline.

As your hips and hands stretch, lean into the idea of releasing stored negative energy and cultivating a fresh feeling of inner strength and security. Stay for 5–10 breaths or longer. To release, place the hands on the floor in front of you and slowly push into a standing forward fold. When you are ready, bend the knees and roll up to standing.

# Middle Back Pain

## THE PAIN OF THE MIDDLE CHILD

Middle back pain tends to get lost until it has reached fever pitch and demands to be noticed! Pain in the middle back may flare up because of strain or injury, prolonged hours of sitting, or what I like to call "losing the jelly in your doughnut." The slightly more scientific definition of this is when the tough outer shell of vertebral discs cracks and the soft part of the discs leaks out, putting pressure on the surrounding nerves. The pain may be localized or spread into buttocks and legs. Fortunately, my personal and professional experience has shown that tremendous improvement can be achieved through yoga! The dynamic duo of strengthening and fostering flexibility comes into play again here.

### 1. Downward Dog (*Adho Mukha Svanasana*)

Downward Dog features prominently in yoga because it serves many conditions. However, it is important that it is practiced properly and with the necessary modifications to meet your body where it is rather than where you want it to be. We must practice from truth not ego—which, ironically, takes practice! When it comes to the middle back, Downward Dog decompresses, stretches, and strengthens the spine in a way that can soothe, refresh, and revitalize those high-pressure points.

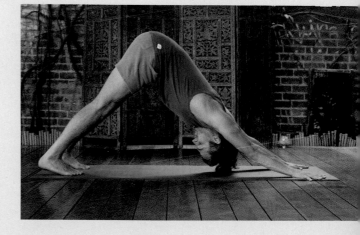

Follow the instructions on page 11. Hold for 5–10 breaths, then bring the knees down and rest in Child's Pose (page 12). Repeat 3 times.

## 2. Extended Side Angle Pose
### (*Utthita Parsvakonasana*)

Warm up for this excellent pose by first doing Downward Dog (page 11). Then, from *Tadasana* (page 9), step your feet wide apart (approximately 4 feet/1.25 meters). Stretch your arms out to your sides at shoulder height with palms facing down. Turn your right foot slightly in toward the center of your body and your left foot out 90 degrees. Imagine a line of chalk that travels straight from your back heel to your front heel. Turn your inner left thigh out so that your left kneecap is in a direct line with the second toe of your left foot. Fire up the leg muscles, drawing them in toward the bones, and as you exhale plant your back heel firmly into the ground—this is the seed from which the pose grows.

Bend your left leg, still tracking the knee over the second toe or center of your ankle. Now you are in Warrior II, but only for a moment! Extending your torso sideways, stretch through your left arm and place your left hand on the floor outside of your left foot—or inside if you have especially tight hips—and use your arm to track your knee over your second toe. In either case, if you can't reach the floor, put your hand on a block or some stable books. If this feels too extreme, place your left forearm on your thigh, being mindful not to collapse onto the thigh but maintaining space around your neck and your shoulders.

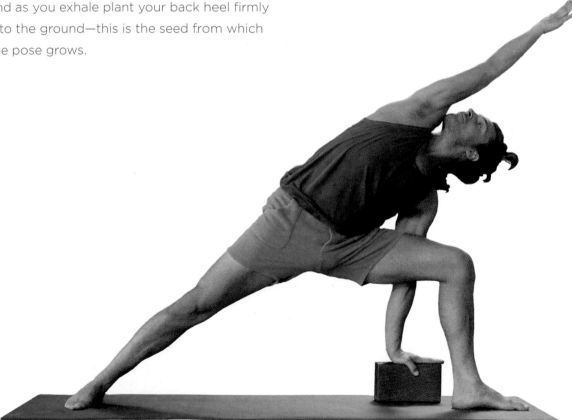

Stretch your right arm directly up and then turn the palm to face the floor and lower the arm to hover a few inches from your right ear. Turn your belly button and chest toward the ceiling and your head toward your right arm. If this aggravates your neck, release it toward the floor and look at your left foot.

Keep pulling your tailbone into your body and press your left elbow and knee against each other to keep the leg tracking safely. Feel the connection between your right outer heel and your right pinky finger, soften your ribs into your body, and breathe. It is important to keep the legs engaged and, after 5–10 breaths, root into the floor with your feet, firm your abdominal muscles, and lift up energetically as though someone is assisting you by pulling your right wrist. Repeat on the other side and then return to *Tadasana*.

### 3. Child's Pose (*Adho Mukha Virasana*)

Child's Pose, which is actually "Downward Facing Hero Pose," is definitely a hero. It is so rich and plentiful in its benefits for body, mind, and spirit that we could just add it onto the end of every one of these mini sequences— and I suggest you do! For our purposes here, we are opening up the back in a gentle yet powerful way and letting the breath soothe muscles, tendons, and nerves. That being said, it is also named after the way many babies sleep, and chances are your flexibility has undergone changes since then, so we must take care in finding the sweet spot.

Follow the instructions on page 12.

**Modification:** If Child's Pose is not possible for you even with added supports, switch to lying on your back hugging your knees into your chest (page 13). This is preferable for those with severe knee trouble or those who find it difficult to relax in Child's Pose.

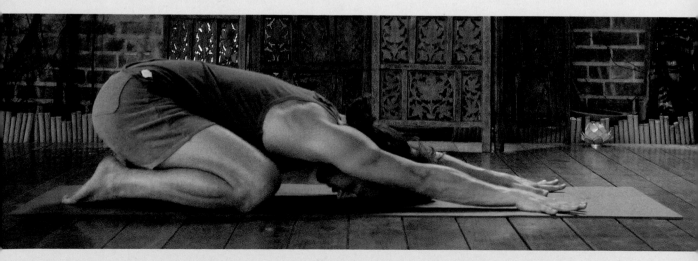

# Lower Back Pain

## YOU ARE NOT ALONE

Every part of the world shares the affliction of back pain by the millions. Of those millions many are suffering chronically, which is widely considered to be three months or longer. The much better news is that yoga really helps and in many cases heals. We know that injury and long hours at a desk or behind the wheel take their toll on the body and in particular the lower back. Back pain also tends to flare up when stress levels are at their peak. So the yoga way would be to kill it (or let's say love it) with kindness. That means strengthen, stretch, and relax. Consistency is key for something chronic, but every little bit does count, so do what you can, when you can, and appreciate yourself for your effort!

### 1. Reclining Hand to Big Toe Pose (*Supta Padangusthasana*)

This pose is as wonderful a stretch for the back as it is fun to say—try it three times fast!—and addresses the hamstrings as well. Since the low back and hamstrings are intimately connected and affect each other, this can only be good.

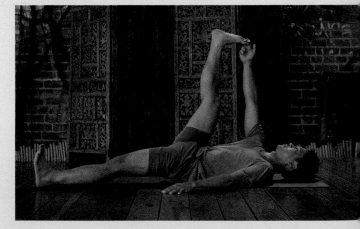

The pose is practiced lying on the floor, which helps to balance and safeguard the back, and using a towel or strap makes the pose possible for those whose toes are out of reach. If you are able to lie flat with your feet against a wall, so much the better, but it's not essential. Press your heels into the wall, or press them away, and press your calves and thighs down toward the ground.

Draw your right knee in to your chest. Both sides of your sacrum and your shoulder blades should be in contact with the floor. Bring the index and middle fingers of your right hand together and wrap them around your right big toe in what is known as "yogi toelock."

Then stretch your right leg straight up toward the sky.

If this is not possible without your shoulder blades or low back losing contact with the floor, place a yoga strap or a towel around your right foot instead of using your fingers. Try to stretch the right leg up at a 90-degree angle, with one hand on each side of your strap and your shoulders and upper back flat to the floor. It may help to slide your hands down the strap until your elbows rest on the floor. If this doesn't work, lower your leg until your upper and lower back regain connection with the floor. Think of your hands as guides and don't grip the strap so tightly that you cause tension in hands or shoulders. Concentrate equally on both legs so that they are equally energized and involved. Hold for 10 breaths or one minute.

To release, draw the right knee back into the chest, remove your strap, and stretch the leg out, pushing the right heel into the wall, or away, along with the left. Repeat on the other side. This pose is dynamite before or after other exercise or activities and also after a long drive or a long day of sitting at a desk.

## 2. Half Locust and Locust Pose
(*Ardha Salabhasana* and *Salabhasana*)

The Locust is a divine strengthening pose for the back, promotes healthy digestion, and elevates the mood. Half Locust is an excellent way to warm up for the full pose.

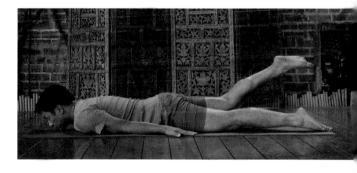

Start by lying on your stomach with your chin on the floor and your arms stretching back alongside your trunk, palms facing up. Lift your right leg as high as you can without straining. Your pelvis and left hip bone remain in contact with the ground. Stretch the leg long and keep it energized all the way through to your toes. If this feels too intense for your lower back, or too strenuous, place your palms on the floor rather than have them facing up. Hold for 5 breaths or 20 seconds, then lower to the ground. Place your forehead on your hands for a few breaths and move to the other side. Repeat this twice on each side.

If you are feeling good, and your back is happy, move into full Locust, but if Half Locust feels like your edge, stay with it for two more rounds on each side. For some people with acute lower back pain or injury to one side of the back, it will actually feel more stable and comfortable to lift both legs in the full pose rather than one at a time in the half version. Some gentle and slow exploration may be needed to settle on the best choice for you.

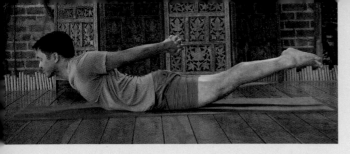

For full Locust, begin on the belly again, place your forehead on the floor, and interlace your hands behind your back with your elbows slightly bent. Roll the shoulder blades toward each other so the front of the shoulders lifts away from the floor. Taking an inhale, lift the whole body until only your hip bones, pelvis, and lower abdomen remain on the ground. Stretch the arms straight back. This version is a wonderful shoulder stretch and heart opener.

Some may find that the hip bones and pelvis lift away from the floor as well. Concentrate on growing long in both directions with your legs extending behind you and your chest reaching forward. Hold for 5 breaths and release, turning your head to one side and listening to your breath. Repeat 3 times. As you repeat, and if your back feels fine, try releasing the interlace of the hands and stretching your arms straight back or even out in front of you with the palms facing each other.

If this pose is not working for your back—that is, you feel discomfort or pain—you can try substituting Cobra Pose (pages 43–44).

## 3. Supine Spinal Twist (*Supta Matsyendrasana*)

And now to the relaxation piece of the puzzle! There is almost nothing as tasty as a supine twist, and you can practically hear your body sigh from deep within as you release and receive. In addition to stretching the back, this pose is excellent for digestion and stretches the neck and chest. If you have an acute injury or severe pain, or have degenerative disc disease, approach the pose with caution and be prepared to place something under your bent knee, such as a block or firm pillow.

Follow the instructions on page 13. If the knee does not reach the floor, you can add the support. If the support is not enough, place it between your knees and roll completely onto your left side, resting your head on your left

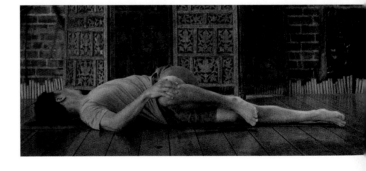

arm, and stay there while your sacrum opens. Hold for 10 breaths and repeat on the other side (**above**). If you are in the version where you are completely on your side, stay for 2–3 minutes before repeating on the other side. Feel your breath flow like water and allow the pose to ripen without effort.

# Lady Trouble

## PMS AND CRAMPS

If irritability, mood swings, bloating, muscle pain, and exhaustion are part of your monthly excursion into all things female, and you are hungry for an exit, a yoga practice may be your golden key to freedom. While it is best (always) to make space for a regular yoga practice to achieve maximum benefits, taking 15 minutes out of your day can work wonders. Turn the lights down, turn the phone off, light a candle if you have one near, and reclaim the beauty of your femininity by nurturing yourself. This body-calming experience can redirect your day before you crash and burn or drown in your own tears of frustration.

### 1. Reclining Butterfly (*Supta Baddha Konasana*)

This is one of my desert-island poses. It's one I cannot live without and hope never to have to! You can take it anywhere. I call it Reclining Goddess. You can practice it lying flat on the floor, or with the support of a bolster or folded blankets or even two blocks or books.

Sit on the floor, spine straight, and bring the soles of your feet together, having placed your support to come right up against your low back. Draw your tailbone underneath you, as if

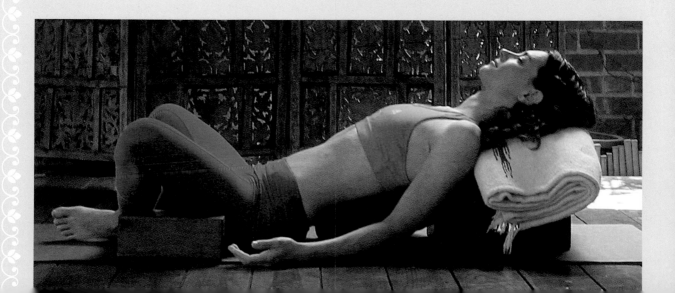

you are smoothing out your skirt to sit down, and then lower your back onto the support. You may want to have a blanket or thin pillow under your head as well. If the stretch feels too much for your hips or knees, place blocks, books, or rolled-up blankets under the outer knees. If the stretch is too extreme for your back, place a block or books under your support where your upper back lands.

Soften into the asana by focusing on your breath in your belly. Take easy, natural breaths and visualize yourself floating in water. By releasing tension in the hips and gently stretching the abdomen, this pose restores harmony to the second, sacral chakra, which is governed by water. It activates and restores our senses of power and comfort, easing anxiety and pacifying an irritable mind. Stay for 5 minutes, or as long as you feel bliss.

## 2. Half Plow Pose (*Ardha Halasana*) and Crocodile Pose (*Makarasana*)

Supported Half Plow pose is a wonderful tonic for bloating, back pain, headache, or sluggishness. However, this pose is best for those who have a regular plow practice or are comfortable with inversions and do not have any neck injuries. If you are new to the pose and enthusiastic about it, try it first with an instructor's supervision. In the meantime, you can skip ahead for Crocodile Pose.

For Half Plow you will need a few props—a chair and two or three blankets that can be folded flat and firm. Place one or two folded blankets beside the chair, touching its legs, and, if you like, one on the seat. Begin by lying on your back with your head and neck off the blankets, but your shoulders and upper back on them, looking up under the chair. Your knees are bent, feet on the floor. When you exhale, press into the floor with your hands and swing your legs over the chair until your thighs rest comfortably on the seat (**below**). You can hold on to the legs of the chair as you adjust this. Keep your head facing up rather than turning your neck from side to side. Relax and let your thighs grow heavy onto the

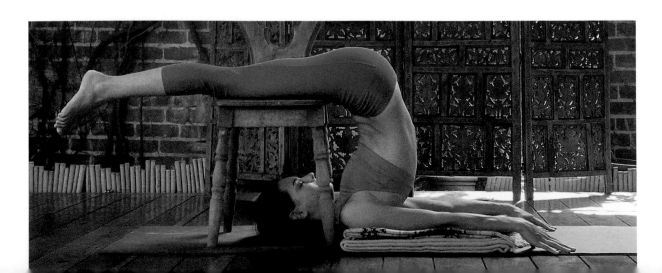

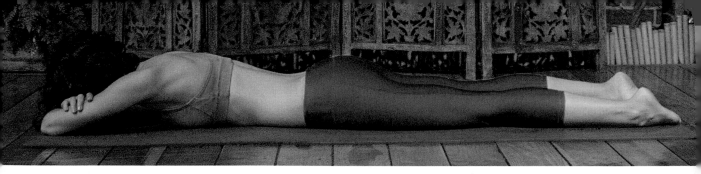

chair. Breathe naturally and enjoy the feeling of support and freedom that comes into your back and hips. Stay for 3–4 minutes. If you feel uncomfortable or nervous in the asana, ease your way out and move on to Crocodile Pose.

**Modification:** If you have a folding chair with an open back, place it sideways against a wall for extra stability and put the blankets in front of the chair. When you swing up, your legs will extend through the chair's back and you can still hold on to its legs as you adjust your position.

For Crocodile Pose, start by lying full out on your stomach. Turn your toes out and let your heels fall in. If this feels very unnatural to you and uncomfortable, do it the other way round so your toes turn in and your heels fall out (**above**). Cross your forearms so that your fingertips come near to your elbows and place your forehead on your forearms. It is especially delicious to place a blanket, bolster, or pillow under your pelvis and hips for a

slight elevation, and also a blanket or small pillow under your feet and ankles. Your chest and head should be slightly elevated. If this is uncomfortable for your chest, you can try resting it on a blanket or pillow as well.

Once you are comfortable, release any gripping or tensing in the muscles, especially in your abdomen, and focus on the breath. If your mind is especially active or anxious, try a variation of Three Part Breath (see page 87). Inhale into your lower back, then Inhale a bit more, focusing on the middle back, and finally inhale to your full capacity with your attention on the back of your heart (upper back). Then exhale and let go of it all. A few rounds of this can lead you into a deep relaxation of body and mind. Stay for 3–5 minutes and, if you prefer, you can turn your head to one side for a couple of minutes and then to the other side. This pose reminds me of a mermaid resting on a beach after a long swim.

### 3. Legs up the Wall or Inverted Action (*Viparita Karani*)

This is one of those one-size-fits-many poses. It is soothing to an aching back, smooths troubled or choppy waters in the low belly known as cramps, and is refreshing overall. Stay 5 minutes or forever! Follow the instructions on page 30.

# Lady Trouble

## FOR THOSE IN THE AGE OF WISDOM

Ah, the price we may pay to enter the golden gates of wisdom. If you have ever felt as though you have been catapulted into a furnace or that your fuse is not only too short but barely even there, you know the prickly edge of menopause. Disrupted sleep, mental fog, sadness, and despair are just a few more symptoms. However, there are many beautiful aspects of the aging process, and when we allow ourselves to be present through the changing terrain, we notice the subtle, and often not so subtle, treasures that are revealed. While a consistent yoga practice can certainly keep our bones dense, muscles strong, and lungs healthy, it may be the sweetness of a deepening compassion for ourselves and all things, which arises from your practice, that becomes the most healing element of all. The following poses are a mini sequence for calming, cooling, and uplifting. For the best results, it is advisable to use these, the PMS sequence, and any others that appeal to you in the book, as often as you can.

## 1. Wide-legged Forward Fold (*Prasarita Padottanasana*)

Begin in *Tadasana* (page 9) with your hands on your hips. Step your feet wide apart with the outer edges of your feet parallel, and your heels aligned with each other. Stretch your arms out wide at shoulder height. It should look as though your wrists track over your ankles (**a**). Bring your hands back to your hips and extend up through your spine and the crown of your head. Inhale and, with a toned core, fold at the hips, maintaining a long spine until you are all the way in to the fold (**b**). Place your hands on the floor (**c**), or on evenly stacked books or blocks, so that when your elbows bend back, your hands are directly underneath them.

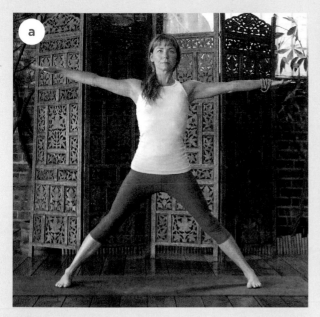

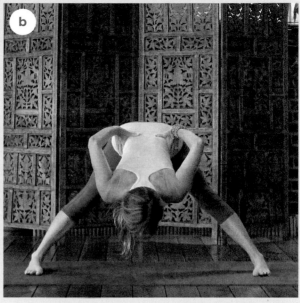

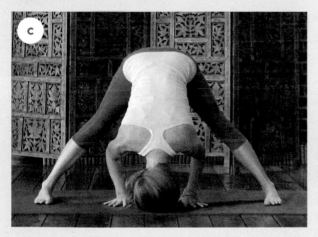

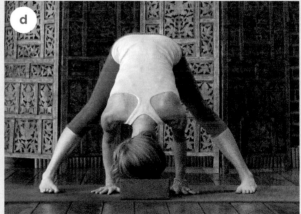

Keep your thighs active and engaged and drop your weight into the balls of your feet. Avoid locking your knees. Allow gravity to pull tension from your neck, shoulders, and even your mind. On your inhales, think of lengthening the spine, and on your exhales drop a little deeper into the fold if you can.

To add a restorative touch, you can place the crown of your head on a support (**d**).

Stay for up to 1 minute. When you lift out of the pose, press strongly into your feet, hug your belly in, and stand up. Come back to *Tadasana*.

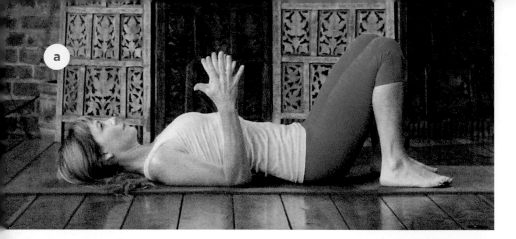

## 2. Bridge Pose (*Setu Bandhasana*) with variations

This restorative heart opener is wonderful for the mood, back, and lungs, to name but a few of its many attributes. Lie on your back with your knees bent and feet parallel. The feet are directly beneath the knees and there is equal pressure on the inner and outer edge of each foot. Bend your elbows as if you are holding a box right over your chest, and puff the chest up while pressing the elbows down (**a**). Now press into the floor with your elbows and your feet and lift your hips into Bridge Pose (**b**).

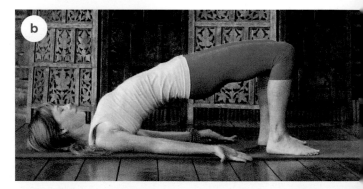

Keep your legs parallel, and if your knees are uncomfortable, try walking your feet 1–2 inches (3–5 centimeters) forward. If your back is uncomfortable, try walking your feet a little bit wider apart. You can keep your arms at your sides, or roll your shoulders underneath you, interlace your fingers, and press your arms down as you lift your torso and chest higher (**c**).

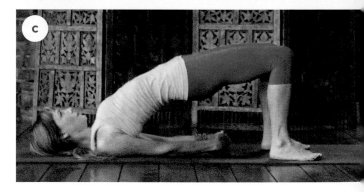

**Variations:** Place a block horizontally, on whichever height is most comfortable for you, directly under your sacrum, which should feel good and supported.

You may want to stay here and enjoy the elevation of hips, heart, and mood, or you may want to take it a step further and lift your legs up straight so that your feet are right over your hips. This takes you into a supported shoulder stand variation (**d**), which is *Setu Bandha Sarvangasana*. If your hamstrings are tight and your legs don't straighten, they can be bent and still track the knees over the hips. Keep your heart lifted and your tailbone down on the block to maintain the backbend and avoid pain from the hard edge of the block in your back. Your arms can be by your sides or interlaced on the far side of the block. Stay 1–3 minutes with your eyes closed or focused softly toward your feet, or concentrate on your third eye with the other two closed.

Another variation is with bolsters or blankets. If you are using blankets, you will need at least three. Fold them firmly in thirds and stack them lengthwise. Sit in the middle of your support and lie back with your head and shoulders coming onto the ground and your legs extending out over the end. If you have an extra blanket, roll it up and place it under your ankles. Relax into your support and into your breath for 3–5 minutes (**e**).

If you are using bolsters, make a "T" with one crosswise and one lengthwise, which goes on top. Sit in the middle of the top bolster and gently lie back with your arms and legs out wide as if you are making a snow angel (**f**). If you need more support for your head, place a folded blanket underneath it.

When you are ready to release either pose, bend your knees and roll off carefully to one side, then push yourself up to a seated position.

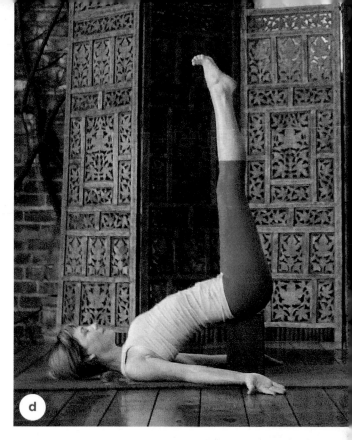

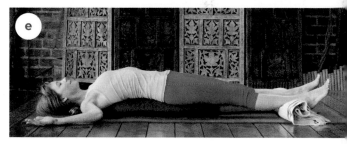

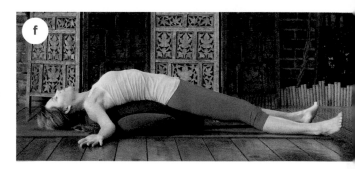

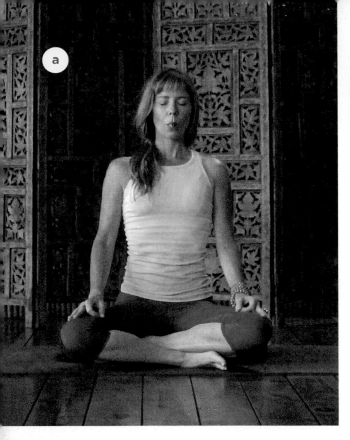

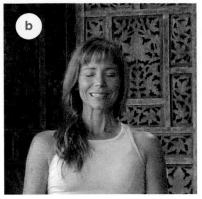

opening, folding it to resemble a straw or tiny taquito. Wait until some saliva has formed and then breathe in through the "straw" (or bird's beak, as the yogis saw it), drinking in the cool moisture (**a**). When you finish inhaling, close your lips and exhale completely through your nose. Continue with the breath for 3–5 minutes if possible.

If you are not genetically predisposed to form a straw with your tongue, you can practice *Sitkari* Breath, which is exactly the same practice but with a variation on the tongue position. For *Sitkari*, gently press your teeth together and open your lips so your teeth are exposed. Draw the moistened air in through the sides of your mouth and exhale through the nose (**b**).

When you have finished the breath practice, stay sitting as you are, and from this calm and cool place, focus your energy toward compassion and appreciation for yourself and your life. It is a gift to be where you are, and one that you richly deserve.

## 3. The Cooling Breath
### (*Sitali* or *Sitkari* Breath)

This natural air-conditioner is perfect for cooling a temper or mitigating a hot flash. It moistens and cools the system and is said to cultivate a love of solitude. Women often find themselves with more solitude as they grow older, and this breath can bring harmony and acceptance during the transition.

Sit cross-legged in *Sukhasana* or *Siddhasana* (page 10) on blankets or a bolster, and place your hands in *Chin Mudra* for focus and grounding by touching the thumb and index finger together, face down on your legs. Take a few deep belly breaths, then form an "O" with your lips and slip your tongue through the

# Bloating

## HAPPENS TO THE BEST OF US

Bloating and digestive troubles are often indiscriminate in their attack. Bloating can occur from what we eat, the way we eat (too much and too fast), and even from swallowing too much air. Stress and anxiety can factor in because they produce cortisol, which inhibits digestion. In stressful times our breathing can be affected, resulting in a shallow breath or holding the breath, and then gulping in too much air. A yoga practice can improve digestion by the way the organs are manipulated in the poses as well as by reducing overall anxiety.

### 1. Hugging Knees to Chest (*Apanasana*) with Supine Twist

Follow the instructions for Hugging Knees to Chest on page 13 (**a**). Relax your abdomen and breathe deeply. Concentrate on relaxing the belly as you breathe. You may feel your abdomen touch your thighs on the inhale and soften into your back as you exhale. Keep your mind on this gentle rhythm. Stay as long as you like, with a minimum of a minute.

Then shift your hips slightly to the left. As you exhale, slowly drop both knees to the right, keeping the knees and ankles stacked. Your chest should face directly up and your shoulder blades keep contact with the floor. Straighten your arms out to the sides at shoulder height. Turn your head to the left for an extra neck stretch. Stay for one minute or longer and then switch sides.

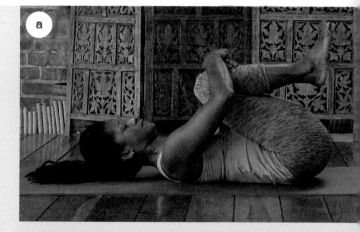

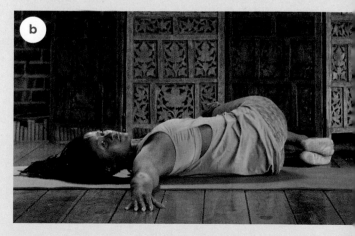

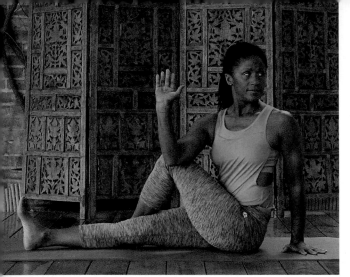

## 2. Half Lord of the Fishes
### (*Ardha Matsyendrasana*)

Sit on the floor with your legs out in front of you. If this already feels like trouble, sit up on a folded blanket to support your low back. Bend your knees so that your feet are on the floor, and slide your right leg under your left. Your right thigh will be on the floor and your left

foot will be squarely on the ground. Hug your left knee to help elongate your spine.

Take your right arm up in the air, as if you were picking the best piece of fruit from the top of the tree, then bend your elbow and bring it down outside of your left knee, as if you were going to take a bite. Keep the hand active. You may enjoy practicing *Jnana Mudra* here, with index and thumb touching on the right hand. Meantime, take your left arm back behind you and press on the floor with your fingertips or palm. If you find it difficult to reach the floor, place a block or books underneath your palm until you can sit comfortably straight. When you inhale, let your abdomen expand as much as it can, and when you exhale, squeeze your navel in toward your spine. Don't force the breath; stay relaxed and alert, concentrating on a full, even breath. Hold for 4–7 breaths, then repeat on the other side.

## 3. Intense Stretch of the West
### (*Paschimottanasana*)

This is a seated forward bend. To start, sit on the floor with your legs straight out in front of you, spine straight, in *Dandasana* (page 9). If your hamstrings or back feel strained, sit on a folded blanket or two. Make sure your legs are active and feet flexed. Then lift your arms, actively stretching straight up, inhale, and as you exhale begin to lower your hands toward your feet. Extend your spine as though you are setting something down just beyond your feet, and when your back begins to round, let your

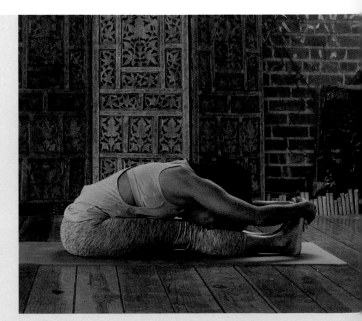

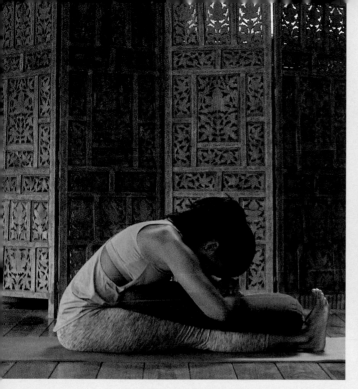

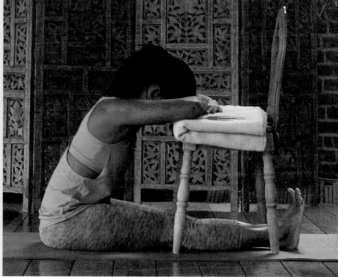

hands land wherever they happen to be, on your knees, shins, or feet. Lengthen and flatten your spine and release your chin so the back of the head remains in line with your spine (**opposite**). Stay for 4–7 breaths.

**Variations:** If this is too strong, widen your legs to make a space the size of a thin slice of pie, but still be sure to stop when your back begins to round.

You can turn the pose into a restorative, which will soothe your nervous system (also helpful when bloated) by adding a bolster or stack of pillows. Either widen your legs to accommodate your support, or keep your legs together and rest the support on top. Extend yourself over the bolster or pillows, stack your hands one on top of the other, and rest your forehead on them (**above**).

A chair is helpful for those who still feel a strain in the hamstrings or back while sitting on blankets. Thread your legs through the legs of the chair and, folding your arms on the seat, place your forehead on your arms. If necessary, add more height by putting a folded blanket on the seat of the chair (**above**). Allow your mind to quieten, feeling your breath and allowing space to enter your belly and your mind.

The last two versions of this pose can be held for 1–3 minutes.

# Tight Hips

## FLEX THE FLEXORS

In my experience, the most frequently requested of all yoga positions are those that open the hips. Perhaps it has something to do with the fact that powerful, and sometimes negative, emotions—often related to the past—are said to be stored in the hips. It is the physical location of the second chakra, *Svadhisthana*, which is the energy center for emotions, and the pelvis is the perfect bowl-like shape to hold them. I also happen to believe that sitting too long, resulting in tight hips, can cause a flood of tears. It's important to let those floodgates open, but it's preferable to do it with flexible hips! Let's stretch ourselves into the present moment with a few poses that will wash your whole bowl clean.

### 1. Low Lunge (*Anjaneyasana*)

There's really nothing like a lunge to get into the front side of the hips known as the hip flexors. For many of us, they suffer from being in the seated "L" position quite often, and this flips that right around.

From Downward Dog (page 11), lift your right leg into the air and, making sure to keep your core engaged, carefully swing your foot forward between your hands. Bring your left knee slowly to the ground and let your knee cap "slide" a bit toward your left foot so you are feeling the pose in that thigh rather than the knee (**a**). If you like, you can have a blanket under your knee for comfort.

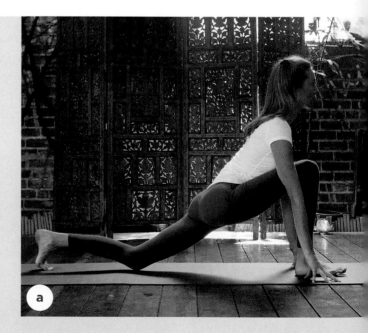

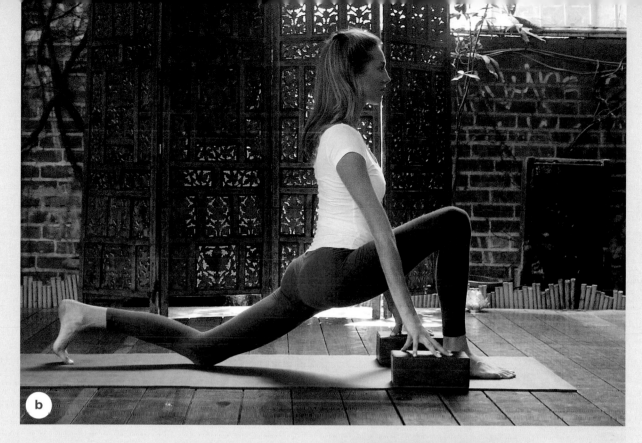

**b**

From here, you can either lift your hands from the floor onto blocks or books (**b**) or raise them overhead (**c**). This choice depends on how stable you feel and how your low back reacts. It is important to maintain active abdominal muscles in this asana if you have a sensitive low back. Repeat on the other leg. Hold for 5–10 breaths on each side and repeat if desired.

**Modification:** If you have a back or shoulder injury, come into the pose from the tabletop position on hands and knees by simply lifting your leg and placing it (or wiggling it) between your hands.

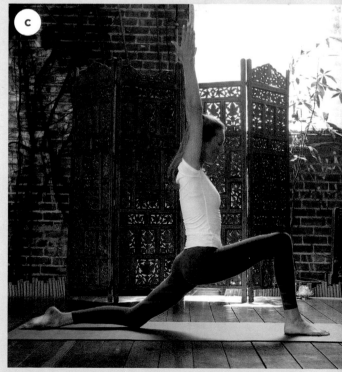

**c**

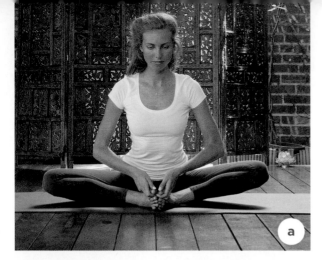

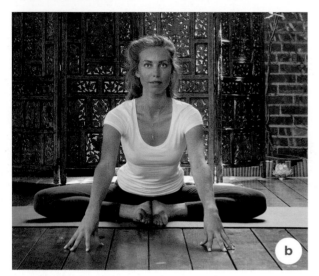

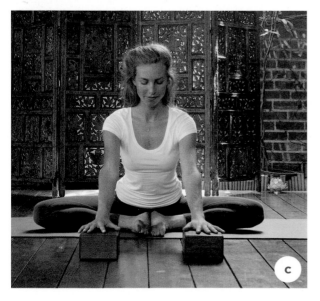

## 2. Butterfly Pose (*Baddha Konasana*)

Also known as Cobbler Pose, this is a favorite and a staple. In addition to the freedom it bestows upon your hips, it serves the reproductive organs in men and women, opens the chest, lengthens the spine, provides relief from sciatica, and lets you gaze into the soles of your feet, which might just be a window to your soul.

In a seated position, bring the soles of your feet together with your knees out to the sides. Wrap your index and middle fingers around your two big toes in yogi toelock and lengthen up through your spine (**a**). Press your feet firmly together with your toes spread apart so you feel your inner thighs wake up, and on an exhale extend forward as far as you can without rounding your back too dramatically. From here you may wish to take your hands out in front of you (**b**) or onto some blocks or books (**c**). Placing the hands in front of you can add a stretch for the shoulders and brings a restorative flavor to the pose. If you stay holding your toes, be sure to curl your big toes slightly in so they don't feel overstretched.

Stay for 1–5 minutes enjoying the sensation of your breath slowly opening and closing the imaginary wings on your back like a butterfly.

### 3. One-legged King Pigeon Pose (*Eka Pada Rajakapotasana*)

I have noticed that pigeons provoke strong responses in people, much like cilantro, and Pigeon Pose is the same. It tends to fall into a love or loathe category. If you land more in the loathe category, try to puff up your chest (like a pigeon) and open your heart, because the benefits of the pose are well worth the struggle. It gets into the psoas and piriformis muscles, which is necessary in order to make headway in clearing the pelvic bowl and truly liberating your hips.

If you are coming from Butterfly Pose (opposite), just swing your right leg behind you and square your hips. Try to move your left leg into a position that is parallel to the front edge of your yoga mat if you are using one. It should resemble a straight horizontal line with your foot flexed (**a**). If this puts a strain on your knee, draw the foot nearer to your pelvis and release the flex. You may want to put a blanket under your left hip if you are sinking to that side and losing the square of your hips. Extend your back leg straight out from the hip and press your toenails into the floor. Your foot should be centered, not sickled. You can stay here propped up on your hands, or you can walk your hands forward into a comfortable "pigeon nap" as long as you maintain the alignment of your hips and legs (**b**, **c**).

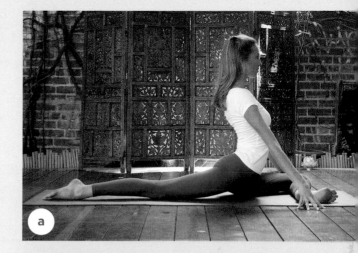

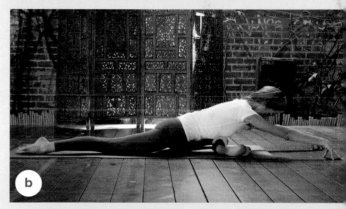

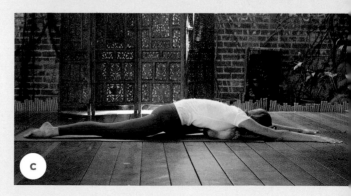

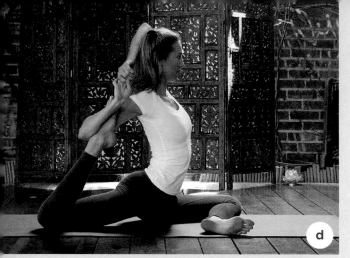

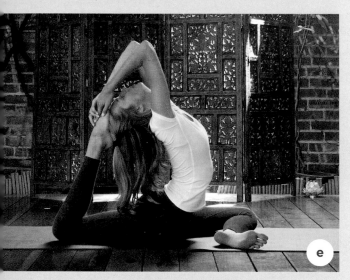

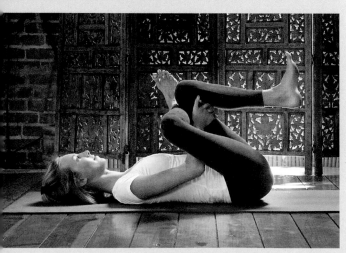

**Variations:** There are a number of variations on your way to the final pose, and you can stop anywhere along the way for your perfect pigeon. If you feel inspired, and your body allows it, you can move into the next step of the pose by bending your right leg and reaching back to clasp your ankle with both hands. You can also clasp your hands behind your head and hook your foot into your right elbow in what some call Mermaid Pose (**d**). Continue to the final pose by stretching your arms up to the sky, bending at the elbows, and taking the sole of your foot to the back of your head (**e**).

**Modification:** Those with knee injuries should practice Reclining Pigeon or Eye of the Needle. For this version, lie on your back with your knees bent and feet on the floor. Cross your right ankle just above your left knee on your left thigh and lift both legs up until you can thread your right hand between your legs and your left hand outside your left leg, clasping them behind your left thigh. Pull the left thigh nearer to you and use your right elbow to press against your right thigh for an even juicier stretch (**below left**). Hold for 5 breaths and repeat on the other side.

# Hamstrings Strung Too Tight

## SCIATICA IN H MINOR

There is almost nothing more frustrating in your asana practice than battling perpetually tight hamstrings, despite your best and most well-intentioned efforts to "restring" them. It can feel as if you are tuning your instrument more than you are getting to play it! Those strings get bound up for many reasons—injury to pelvic alignment, overload of exercise (yes, that can happen!), and too much work, to name a few. It is also possible that the sensation of tight hamstrings or injury is caused by compression of the sciatic nerve, which stems from the discs in the low vertebrae. Stretching through yoga is a key component in getting your legs to sing again, but it must be done carefully or you can create more tension than you release.

Since the hips, pelvis, and back have a direct effect on the hamstrings (and vice versa), I suggest you practice the poses from the hips and low back sections of the book before the hamstring poses as often as you can. Never force the hamstrings, and always breathe and relax into the stretch. Now, let's hear from the string section, shall we?

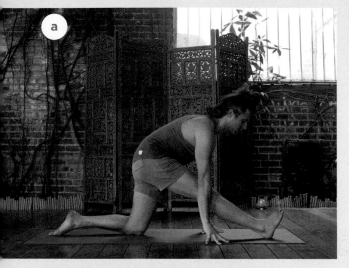

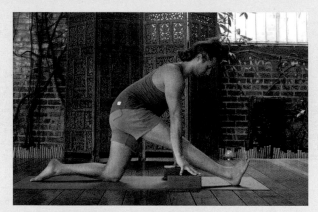

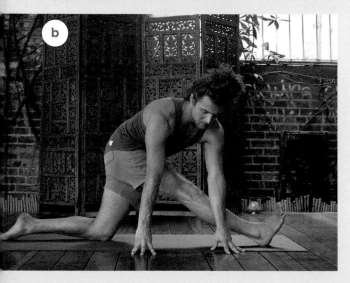

# 1. Half Monkey God Pose
## (*Ardha Hanumanasana*)

This pose delivers quite a punch, and most likely will not feel as if you are monkeying around. You may need a blanket under the knees. Begin on hands and knees and step your right foot forward between your hands. Keep your hands on fingertips underneath your shoulders and straighten your right leg out in front of you so that the heel is on the floor and the toes are stretching up toward the ceiling (**a**). If you are hunched over, or you can't reach the floor, have blocks or books under your hands (**left**). Keep the right foot flexed and do not lock the right knee. Your left hip should be above your left knee and your hips should be square. Engage your right thigh. Hold the pose for 3–5 breaths, then walk both hands outside of the right thigh for a light twist for 3–5 breaths before switching sides (**b**).

The breath is important in every asana, but especially so here. If you concentrate on allowing the breath to be the main focus once you have aligned yourself in the pose, your body will relax into the asana and create space for transformation rather than more tension in an already tense area. Let gravity be your friend here.

**Variation:** Another technique to explore in these poses is to contract the muscles for 3 breaths, stay in the pose, and follow that by relaxing the muscles for 3 breaths. In any case, the breath is essential to making beautiful music.

## 2. Gate Pose (*Parighasana*)

This great hamstring pose also offers an invigorating side stretch. Kneel on the floor or a blanket with your hands on your hips and stretch your right leg out to the right. Either point the toe, placing the foot on the floor, or place a block under the foot for support. Align your right heel with your left knee and keep your left hip directly over the left knee. Your right kneecap is facing directly up. Your left hip bone can come slightly forward of your right, but keep your belly button facing directly out in front of you.

Stretch your arms up and widen them out to the sides (**a**). Turn your palms facing down. As you inhale, stretch your right arm out over your right leg toward your right foot, and lower your hand as you exhale. It may go to the floor, a block, or your leg (**b**). Stretch your left arm up and move it over your left ear. Look up at your left elbow if your neck allows (**c**).

If you feel a strain in the back of your right knee, you can set a block up under your right calf and press your calf into it. This will take the pressure off of the knee and allow you to relax into the asana. Hold for 3–5 breaths and then lift from the left arm, by pressing down through the legs. Bring the right leg in and either sit back on your heels for a few moments or go straight to the other side.

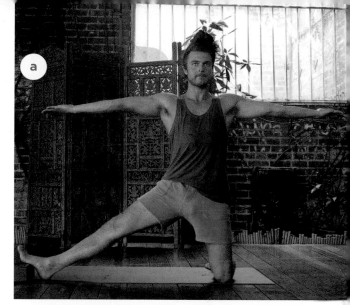

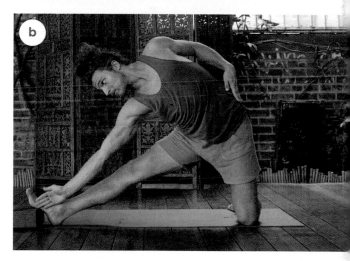

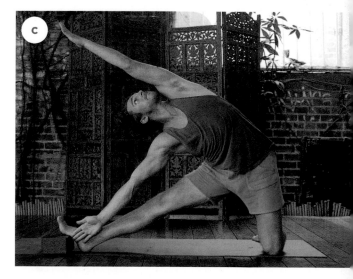

### 3. Intense Side Stretch (*Parsvottanasana*)

First, have your support ready—blocks or evenly stacked books—in case you are not able to reach the floor in this pose. Stand in *Tadasana* (page 9) and, on an inhale, step your feet wide apart (approximately 4 feet/1.25 meters), parallel to each other. With your hands on your hips, turn your left foot to the right by 45–60 degrees and your right foot to the right by 90 degrees. Swivel your torso to face completely to the right. If you feel as if you are on a tightrope and balance is tricky, move your right foot a couple inches to the right (**a**).

Now, facing squarely in the direction of the right leg, inhale and let your tailbone descend as you lift up through the crown of the head. Press firmly into your left heel, exhale, and lower your torso until it is parallel to the ground. Release your hands to the floor or your support, keeping your arms straight (**b**).

Keep pressing firmly down through your legs like the roots of a tree clinging to the earth, and line your right kneecap to the center of your leg and facing up. Squeeze the legs toward each other, but let the right femur grow heavy toward the earth. Fold nearer to your leg if you can, bending at the elbows if necessary, and relax the head and neck (**c**). Otherwise, extend the back of your neck and head, keeping them aligned with your spine and your face pointing toward the floor. Stay focused on keeping your hips square and your breath flowing. When you feel that you've held the stretch long enough, repeat for the other side of the body.

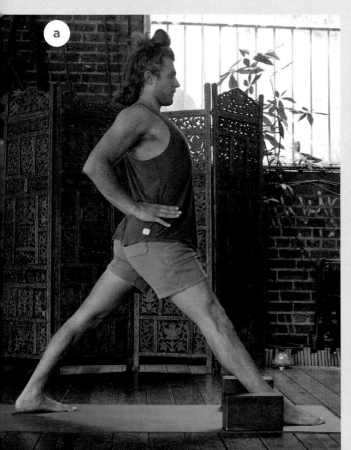

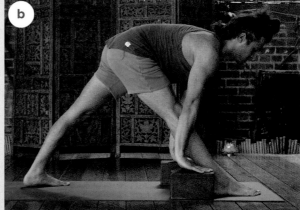

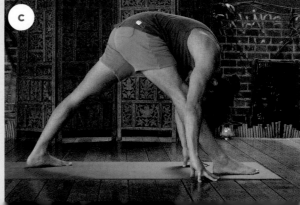

# Thighs and Knees

## YOU'RE ONLY AS GOOD AS YOUR KNEES

Well, fortunately this lyric from a song I love does not adequately describe your worth from a yogic perspective, but it does make a good point, and the knees are worth tending to before they raise a ruckus. These precious shock absorbers bear the brunt of much of our life experience. Being active is essential for good health, but activity plays out in the joints and can leave them prone to a variety of sensitivities. If through injury, arthritis, or developmental issues your knees are not pleased, take heart—there is hope. In the case of the knees, what strengthens often heals, but a fair dose of stretch for the quadriceps is a main ingredient. Prevention and healing often look the same in yoga where the knees are concerned.

### 1. Chair Pose (*Utkatasana*)

Sitting in a chair and sitting in Chair Pose are two very different experiences! Start in *Tadasana* (page 9) with the feet together and parallel to each other, spine straight, and kneecaps lifted. You may be more comfortable with your heels slightly apart and toes touching. Try both ways and see which fits.

Bend the knees and sweep the arms straight up in front of you until your biceps are alongside your ears. Rock into your heels a bit. Spread your toes and place them down on the mat with space between each toe. Keep the weight in the heels while still pressing into the

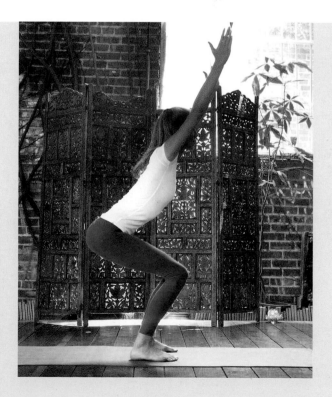

balls of the feet. Let your shoulders drop away from your ears (avoid the shrug position) and keep the arms vibrantly straight. Contract your navel toward your spine to protect the back. You should have a natural and comfortable curve in your lumbar spine, but not an exaggerated arch. Hold for 5 breaths, then push into the earth with strong legs and stand up in *Tadasana*. Repeat 3–5 times.

**Modifications:** If your shoulders are tight, it may be better for you to spread your arms farther apart to take the pressure out of your neck and trapezius (the big triangular muscle at the top of the back). Another option is to hold the arms in front of you at shoulder height, palms facing up. Above all, don't strain or tense up in the shoulders or you will do more harm than good.

If having your legs together with the knees touching does not work for your body type, or you are pregnant, you can start with your feet hip-width apart. Don't let your knees fall in when you sit. Keep them tracking over your toes.

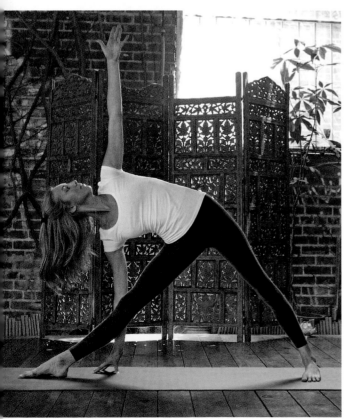

## 2. Triangle Pose (*Trikonasana*)

The holy trinity of triangle! A mystic of a pose! And one that, to me, really feels like yoga. It is rooted, expansive, and heart expanding, and just happens to be good for aligning and strengthening the knees.

Start in *Tadasana* (page 9), place your hands on your hips, and step your feet wide apart (approximately 4 feet/1.25 meters). Turn your left heel to the left slightly and your right foot 90 degrees to the right. Stretch your arms out to the sides at shoulder height with the palms facing down.

As you inhale, reach out over your right toe tips with your right hand and extend your torso out over the right leg. Exhale and place your right hand on your leg, a block, or the floor (**left**). You can have the hand inside or

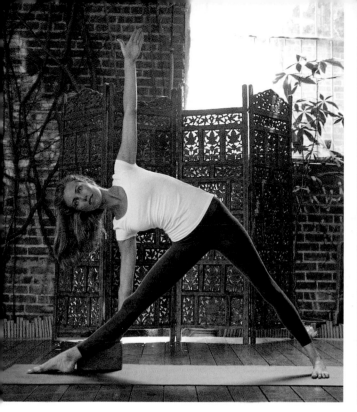 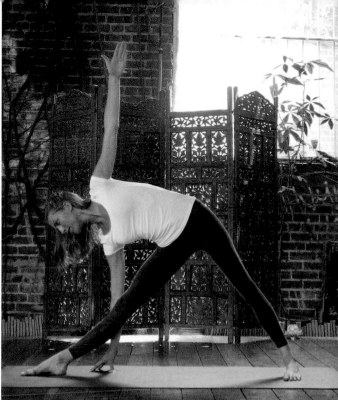

outside of the right foot, as long as you are able to keep your right hand under your right shoulder and extend both sides of your waist toward the right. Engage your thighs and track your right knee over your shin bone and down to your second right toe. Your left arm is directly over your left shoulder and your focus point (*drishti*) is your left thumb. If possible, don't bend the neck to the side, but keep it extending directly out from your spine. Avoid the broken flower syndrome here with your head hanging sadly to the side. Hold for 2–5 breaths, come up with a strong core and legs, and repeat on the other side.

**Modifications:** If your neck is uncomfortable, look straight ahead (**above left**, shown with a block), or look down toward the floor instead of up at your thumb, and let your neck bend (**above**). This is a safer angle to release the neck. If the back of the right knee feels strained or looks or feels hyperextended, bend the knee a tiny bit. If this doesn't release pressure on the knee, place a block under your right calf at an angle and press your calf into the block to keep it stable. This is a great way to strengthen your quadriceps and knees without applying too much pressure to the joint. You can also play with lifting your toes up on either or both feet to engage the legs more.

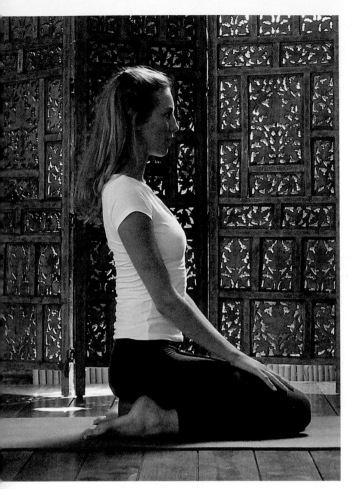

### 3. Hero Pose (*Virasana*)

Be your own hero with *Virasana*. This noble asana lengthens the quads, which can release pressure on the knees. Begin in the tabletop position on hands and knees, then bring your knees together and your feet a little wider than your hips. Reach back with both hands and pull your calf muscles toward your feet, opening a pocket of space behind the knees. Slowly sit back between your feet, until your rear is on the floor. Make sure that the top of the foot is on the floor and all ten toenails are touching the ground. Using your fingers, spread the toes apart. Place your hands on your thighs or take the Mudra of Contemplation, with your right hand under your left across the body and your thumbs touching in a circle. Pick a focus point or close your eyes and take the *drishti* within. Begin with 5–10 breaths and work up to 5 minutes.

**Modifications:** It may be clear that this sitting position is not going over well with your knees! If so, sit on a block, a stack of books, or firmly folded blankets. If the knees are still uncomfortable, roll up a blanket or yoga mat and place it behind the knees to create more space in the joints. If your ankles hurt, place a blanket underneath your feet.

# Oh My Aching Feet

## AND CRUNCHY ANKLES!

If you spend a lot of time standing, have tight or weak ankles, suffer from plantar fasciitis (thickening of a band of tissue under the sole of the foot), have fallen arches, are pregnant, or simply have tuckered-out feet, these yoga remedies can put the spring back in your step. These poses are for strengthening and stretching, but if your feet simply need a break, cool them off with Legs up the Wall Pose (page 30).

### 1. Eagle Pose or "King of the Birds" (*Garudasana*)

Garuda—an eagle deity—has been identified with the "all-consuming fire of the sun's rays," and you may feel as though you are being consumed in this electric asana. Be assured that it will strengthen and stretch the ankles while you sharpen your balance and focus, among other benefits.

Stand in *Tadasana* (page 9) and bring your hands to your hips. Bend your knees slightly and shift your weight to your right foot as you cross your left thigh over your right. Point your left toe and wrap it around behind your right calf, hooking it into your lower calf, so that you are balancing on your right foot.

Stretch your arms wide to the sides and inhale (**a**).

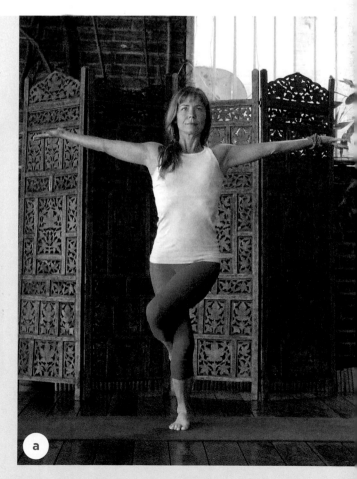

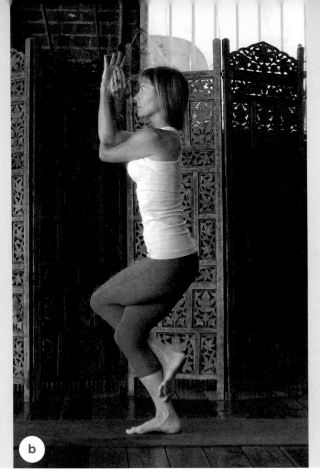

b

As you exhale, cross your arms in front of you with the right arm going over the left. Bend at the elbows, move the backs of the hands toward each other until they pass, placing the left fingers into the center of your right palm. Lift the arms to shoulder height and away from you (**b**).

Hold the pose with steady breath and gaze for 3–5 breaths or 15–30 seconds, before releasing into *Tadasana* and switching sides.

**Modifications:** If you cannot wrap your foot around your calf, concentrate on squeezing the upper legs together and let the foot get as near to the standing leg as possible. If the shoulders are preventing you from crossing your hands, just go as far as you can and keep the fingers energized.

## 2. Raised Lunge or Horseriding Pose (*Utthita Ashwa Sanchalanasana*)

From Downward Dog (page 11) or tabletop position, step the right foot between the hands. Extend the left leg behind you, balancing on the ball of the foot. Your right knee is directly over your right foot and your hands or fingertips are on the floor beneath your shoulders. "Scissor" or "hug" the inner thighs toward each other without moving your feet, and pull your belly button in (**a**).

Reach your arms out in front of you and continue lifting them up—imagine that you are placing the sun back in the sky. Bring your arms alongside your ears, keeping the

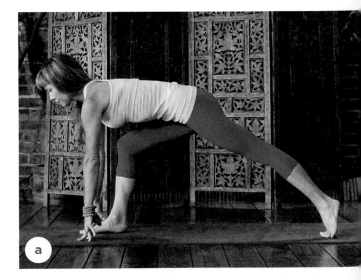

a

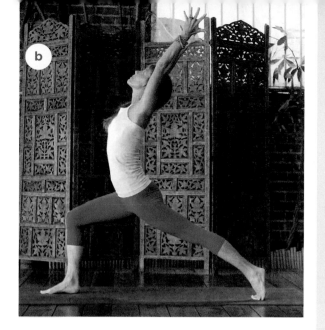

b

abdomen strong and your breath fluid. Lift your gaze slightly higher than eyeline and let the light pour in (**b**). Hold for 3–5 breaths, then release the arms to the floor and repeat on the other side.

**Modifications:** If you have an ankle injury or this is too strenuous, keep your hands on the floor or blocks. If you place the knee of the extended leg on the floor, you will get a subtler stretch with no pressure (**below**). As an alternative to this pose, you could practice Garland Pose (page 48).

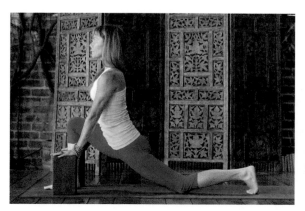

## 3. Thunderbolt Pose *(Vajrasana)*

This is a precursor to Hero Pose and also a wonderful meditation and pranayama pose. In addition to stretching the feet and ankles, it produces a good stretch for the quads and knees, and aids digestion. Sit on your shins with your sitting bones on the soles of your feet. Your feet should be centered, with all ten toenails on the floor. Soften your ribs into your body and keep your spine straight. Place your hands on your thighs either palms down or palms up, with the thumb and index fingertips together in *Jnana Mudra*. Relax the muscles of your face and open to the power and strength of your spine. This position is especially useful for connecting with the *Sushumna Nadi*, which is the central channel of energy in the body and is said to run parallel to the spine. Connect with your vital life force as you breathe into the eternally present moment. Stay 1–5 minutes or longer.

**Modifications:** If your feet and ankles are uncomfortable on the floor, place a folded blanket under the shins and feet. If your knees are unhappy, place a thinly folded blanket between your seat and your legs. Add more support there as necessary.

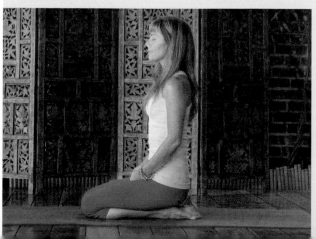

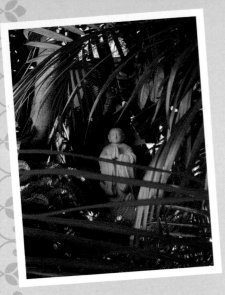

**PART 2**

# Remedies for the Mind

WHO *IS* RUNNING THIS SHOW?

### Mind

"(In a human or other conscious being) the element, part, substance, or process that reasons, thinks, feels, wills, perceives, judges, etc.; intellect or understanding, as distinguished from the faculties of feeling and willing; intelligence"

### Thought

"The product of mental activity; that which one thinks; the capacity or faculty of thinking, reasoning, imagining, etc."

### Consciousness

"The state of being conscious; awareness of one's own existence, sensations, thoughts, surroundings, etc.; the thoughts and feelings, collectively, of an individual or of an aggregate of people"

Oh, these beautiful minds! You can get a headache thinking about the mind, but it is a glorious thing to ponder and possess—the most magnificent technology yet created, and so much more than that. The mind has the mysterious ability to observe itself being observed. Your mind can think a thought, and know it's thinking, and at the same time have trouble distinguishing between reality and a passing fancy or intrusive thought. The power of the mind over our life experience is infinite. We are living and perceiving through the judgments, opinions, data analysis, and stored memories of the mind. If we can compassionately direct ourselves toward the liberating moment of the present, we can take a breath of fresh air and clarity. We can create our own reality in the moment in a way that is not bound by comparison and overthinking. We can finesse our perception and make conscious choices that lead to beliefs that serve us—beliefs are simply thoughts that we practice.

Is the mind friend or foe? So much in the practice of yoga is about stilling or quietening the mind, rising above it, that you would think the mind was simply in the way of achieving any sort of peace and freedom. While there is some truth to this, the mind can also be viewed as a wild and majestic horse that simply needs to be loved (not broken) into calmness so that its own reckless energy doesn't consume it. The energy of the mind is so strong that it has trouble sitting still in the present and constantly travels back and forth from past to future, searching for what is already available right here in the now—comfort, inspiration, and peace.

In yoga, we use the body to corral the mind to the task at hand. "Pay attention to your feet on the floor!" When it has tired of trying to think of other things while paying attention to breath and physical sensation, we are able to wrangle it gently, to soothe and settle it right into our own laps as we meditate. It is then that we experience the oneness or unity that the skittish mind so often persists in keeping just outside of our grasp. If we can accept what is—in the world, in our lives, in the moment—even though we may not like it, much of the struggle is gone. In the absence of struggle, the mind's true and productive capabilities shine and the world becomes illuminated.

We will use the asanas, breath, and meditation to encourage, persuade, and relax the mind into the eternally present moment from which all is possible, and where all exists. I strongly recommend that you meditate at the end of each sequence for 3–15 minutes. Developing a consistent meditation practice is truly transformational. Keep it simple, focus on your breath, and sit quietly.

*"To rise above the modifications of your mind, when you cease your mind, when you cease to be a part of your mind, that is yoga."*
Patanjali

# Anxiety

## SMALL STEPS FOR A BIG FEELING

In small doses, anxiety that is predominantly situational is a normal part of life, but it can become a tidal wave with an extreme undertow, leaving you struggling to keep your head above water. The inner turmoil, muscular tension, mental exhaustion, and general nervousness that are characteristic of anxiety are no fun in any size. Yoga works beautifully for assuaging anxious moments in life; and as part of a comprehensive treatment for more severe situations, it is a powerful supplement. The release of adrenaline and cortisol, which is associated with the fight or flight response, can take a toll on the body while the mind struggles to stay in check. Practicing yoga can slow down the body's response and aid the overworked adrenal glands. This is a salve to the immune system as well as your nerves.

### 1. Tree Pose (*Vrksasana*) with *Hakini Mudra*

Balancing poses, such as Tree, draw us into the present moment and away from the distracting chatter of the mind. It is challenging enough to stand on one foot like a mighty sequoia, let alone engage with the churning of your psyche while doing so!

Stand in *Tadasana* (page 9) and choose a focus point (*drishti*). Feel all four corners of each foot placed evenly and firmly upon the earth (**a**). Bring your hands to your hips and shift your weight to the right foot.

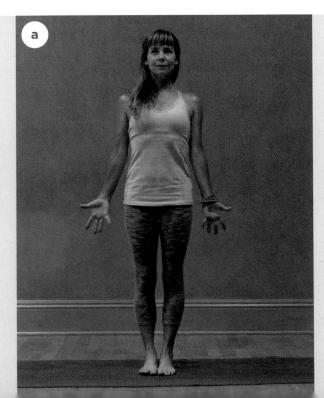

Lift your left leg, bending the knee until you can reach down for your ankle without bending over too significantly. Once you have grasped your ankle, place it on the upper inner right thigh with your toes pointing toward the floor. Keep pressing your inner right foot down to stay rooted. Rotate your inner left thigh out as much as you can to open that left hip.

Now bring all five fingertips of each hand together, leaving the palms apart (*Hakini Mudra*), and hold directly in front of your heart. Keep a firm but light touch. This mudra brings your attention to the moment, boosts memory, balances the opposing energies in the body, and helps us connect to the third eye, developing our intuition, all of which can produce greater clarity and calm (**b**).

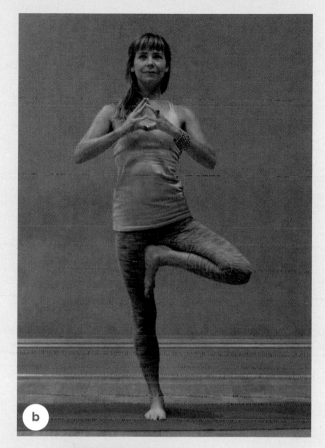

Tree Pose has many other elevating aspects that are liberating for body and mind. It's a deep hip release (let go!), builds strength and endurance (focus!), and increases flexibility (don't be too rigid!), which are all essential for inner peace. If you can detach from the ego and the need to stay up by letting your breath rustle through your pose like the wind in the leaves of the tree, it can evolve into a peak experience. Stay for 5–10 breaths or until you feel the urge to move, and release into *Tadasana* before you switch sides.

**Variation:** You could add an extension of your arms upward for the last few breaths if you feel inspired (**right**). This arm variation is very uplifting and may surprise you by affording you more balance! When you finish the breaths or feel ready, release into *Tadasana* before you switch sides.

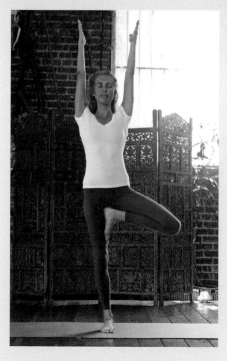

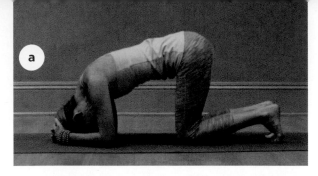

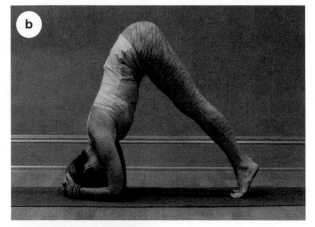

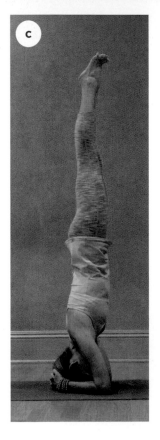

## 2. Headstand (*Salamba Sirsasana*)

Headstand may not be for everyone—those with head or neck injuries, detached retina, or early stage or high-risk pregnancy, for example—but it is considered "King of the Asanas" and is worth exploring if you are able. It can refresh your perspective and quieten the mind. I strongly suggest that if you are new to the pose, you practice with a wall behind you, and if you have an experienced yogi in your life who knows how to "spot," enlist their help. For alternative poses, see below.

Use a blanket or mat to cushion your arms and head. From hands and knees, place your forearms on the floor with your elbows under your shoulders, and lace your fingers together. Place the crown of your head on the floor between your hands. If you are new to the pose, clasp your hands, pressing the back of your head up against the inner wrists. More experienced practitioners can open their hands and nestle the back of the head into the open palms (**a**).

Lift your hips (think Dolphin or Downward Dog, pages 134 and 11) and walk your feet in, creating a V shape. Pull your shoulder blades into your back and keep lengthening your torso to avoid putting too much pressure on the head or shoulders (**b**). Push against the floor with your arms and as you inhale begin to lift both your legs. You can bend the knees or lift them both straight up using your core strength. If you are working with a spotter, or even at the wall, take one leg up and with a light push send the other up to meet it. This is an option, provided you are not jumping into the pose in a way that puts strain on your neck or causes your foundation to shift or collapse.

Once you are up, think of being in an inverted *Tadasana* (page 9), with the belly button as the center of the pose. Align the arches of your feet with your hip bones, and soften your fingers and jaw. Reach up through active legs, flex your feet or press through the balls of the feet, relax, and breathe (**c**).

If you are new to headstand, stay for a few breaths and then rest in Child's Pose for 1–2 minutes (page 12). Gradually add a few breaths to each practice until you are comfortable with 3 minutes in headstand. For seasoned yogis, hold the pose for up to 10 minutes, as long as you don't feel pain.

If headstand is not for you, try Shoulder Stand (pages 35–36) or Legs up the Wall (page 30) instead.

### 3. *Hansi Mudra* and *Dirga* Breath

*Hansi Mudra* promotes a feeling of courage and fearlessness and is wonderful for anxious minds and feelings of loneliness or isolation. Sit comfortably in a seated pose on the floor or on a chair. Bring the thumb, index, middle and ring finger together on each hand. Extend your pinky. Place the back of the hands on your thighs or knees. Close your eyes, if that feels comfortable.

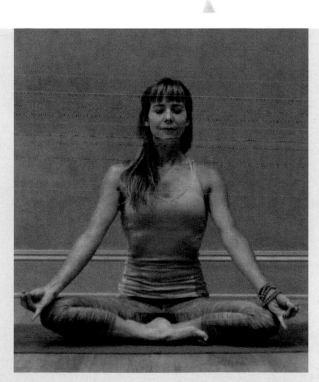

Now begin *Dirga* Breath. Inhale into the bottom of your belly, then your solar plexus, finishing the breath in your chest. You may find it helpful to visualize filling a glass with water from the bottom to top. Pause briefly when you have filled your glass and then exhale from the upper chest, solar plexus, and finally bottom of the belly as if you were pouring the water from the glass. Continue with *Dirga* (also known as Three Part Breath) for 1–3 minutes.

# Lack of Focus

## SORRY, COULD YOU REPEAT THAT?

It can happen any time, anywhere, and often at the worst possible moment. Your mind wanders in every direction but where you need it to stay right now. Our ability to focus can be affected by many things—lack of sleep, stress, and anxiety, for example. Lack of focus and memory loss are also related to depression and certain diseases and conditions, and can be a part of the aging process. However, yoga and meditation have been proven to have a positive and regenerative effect in many cases. As stated by the yogic sage Patanjali in the Yoga Sutras, "*Yoga chitta vritti nirodha*," which translates as, "Yoga is the reduction of fluctuations of the mind." Here are a few techniques for wrangling that magnificent mind of yours and sharpening your focus when you need it.

### 1. *Tadasana* with *Anjali Mudra*

Stand up tall with your feet together and your arms extended energetically by your sides in *Tadasana* (page 9). Balance on each foot equally from the inner to the outer and from the ball to the heel. Firm your legs. Set a focus point (*drishti*) and take 5 breaths through your nose. On an inhale, raise your arms overhead and bring the palms together (**a**), then bring them down the front of your body to your heart center, the middle of the chest (**b**). This is *Anjali Mudra*. Maintain your gaze (*drishti*) for 5 more breaths.

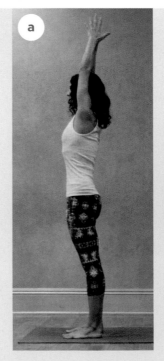
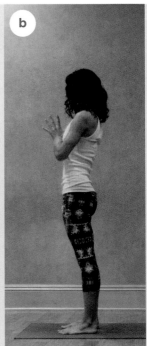

## 2. Warrior II (*Virabhadrasana II*)

Follow the instructions on page 98 to come into Warrior II. Engage your abdominals and hold for 3–5 breaths. On an inhale, lift out of the pose and rest your hands on your hips. Turn your feet to the other side and repeat.

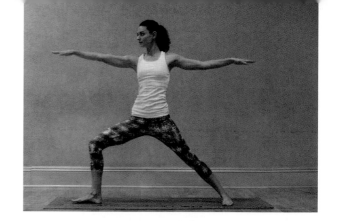

## 3. Alternate Nostril Breathing (*Nadi Shodhana*)

This pranayama technique clears the two main energy channels of the body and balances the hemispheres of the brain, which can result in greater energy and focus.

Sit comfortably and position your left hand, facing up or down, with the thumb and index finger touching in *Jnana* or *Chin Mudra* (*Jnana* is up, *Chin* is down). Otherwise rest your hand comfortably on your thigh. Place your right thumb to your right nostril with the index and middle fingers folded into your palm. Inhale deeply through your left nostril. At the top of your inhale place the ring finger of your right hand over your left nostril, gently pinching the nose and pausing the breath. Then release your thumb and exhale through the right nostril. Inhale through the right nostril, close both, and exhale through the left. This is one cycle.

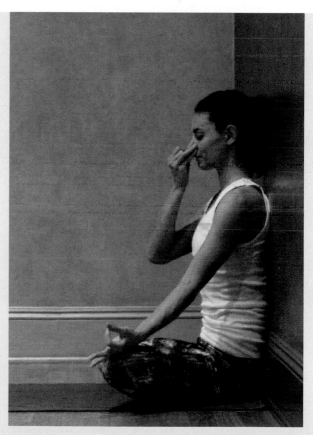

Continue with 5–10 cycles, maintaining a consistent length between the inhale, the pause, and the exhale. It may be helpful to use a count such as 5 in, 5 hold, 5 out. Enjoy the bright boost this powerful practice will give you.

# Impatience

## WHAT'S THE RUSH?

The feeling of impatience tends to be as unsavory for the person feeling it as for anyone else in the vicinity. It may play out as road rage, arguments with family, grumpy parenting, or a nagging feeling of never having enough time. Impatience fosters the idea that things, or people, are standing in your way, preventing you from achieving your goals. The size of the goals may fluctuate, but the edgy feeling of things being in your way can seem big and persistent. At times the sound of life's clock ticking can be deafening, and it can leave us feeling powerless and grasping for control. When we practice trust and contentment (*Santosha*), we can develop a rapport with time and circumstances that is more amicable and spacious. This does your blood pressure a world of good, as well as your heart, your head, and your relationships.

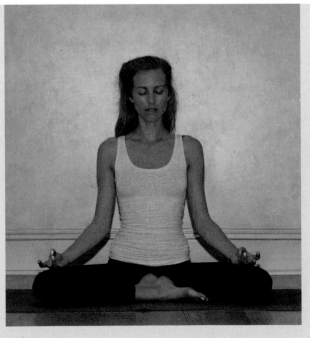

### 1. Meditation with Mudra for Contentment

Once, when I was young, I eagerly opened a fortune cookie only to discover that "The reward of patience is patience." I felt gypped and impatient. Years later I came to appreciate it greatly. When we practice meditation, we often encounter the greatest of obstacles—the mind. If you are new to meditating, the mere act of sitting quietly is likely to highlight your lack of patience, rather than it seeming like the path to freedom that it is. It's a perfect opportunity! The reward for staying with it will indeed be greater patience, starting with yourself.

Sit comfortably cross-legged in *Sukhasana* or *Siddhasana* (page 10), or on a chair, with your spine straight. Women should touch their right thumb to their right middle finger and their left thumb to their pinky for *Santosha Mudra*. Men should reverse the fingers. Concentrate on following your breath as it moves in your body. It may help to count your breaths, such as 4 counts for an inhale and 6 for an exhale. If your mind is especially overactive and you find counting frustrating, listen to the sounds around you. Observe them without commentary. Practice active listening without agenda. Allow yourself whatever experience comes forth. There is no right way as you explore being present for 3–5 minutes.

**Variation:** Another option for focusing and calming the mind is to say silently as you inhale "*San*" and silently as you exhale "*tosha*," with the intention of embracing the present from a place of acceptance.

## 2. Head to Knee Pose (*Janu Sirsasana*)

Sit on the floor in *Dandasana* (page 9)—spine straight, legs straight out in front of you, feet flexed. Reach behind your inner left knee and pull your leg back, placing your left foot into your right inner thigh near your groin (**a**). If this is painful for your left knee, slide the left foot down your right leg until it feels more comfortable.

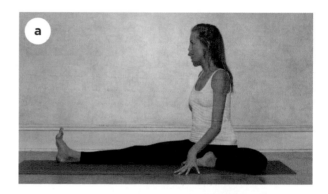

Sit tall and lift your arms overhead (**b**). Then stretch your torso over your extended leg. Line your belly button up with the center of your right thigh. Your hands may be on either side of your right leg or clasped on the sole of your foot. Inhale, and lift and lengthen your spine before letting your head gently bow toward your chest, exhaling and settling into the pose. Keep your right leg active with the toes pointing up (**c**).

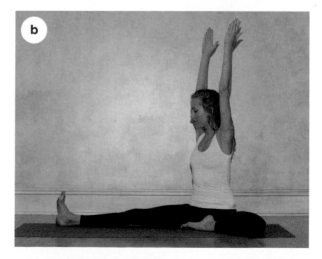

Breathe and let go for 5–10 breaths before switching sides. Concentrate on finding contentment with things as they are in this moment.

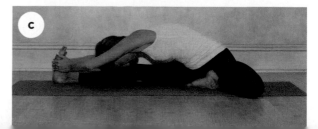

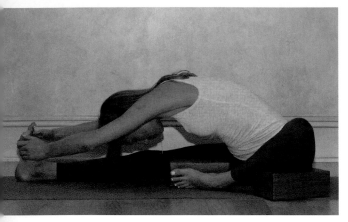

**Modifications:** Sit on a blanket if your low back feels tender or tight. If your left hip is tight, place a block under your outer left knee. If you are experiencing knee pain on the left side, place a block between your left foot and inner right thigh.

**Variation:** For a more restorative version of the pose, place a bolster or folded blankets on your right leg and fold over the support. Rest your forehead on the support.

### 3. Left Nostril Breathing (*Chandra Bhedana*)

This is also called Moon Breath. Sit cross-legged on the floor, spine tall, or on a chair, left hand relaxing on your thigh or with thumb and index fingertips meeting in *Jnana Mudra*. Fold the index and middle finger of your right hand into your palm. Place your right thumb on your right nostril and inhale through the left. Then place your ring finger on your left nostril and pause for a few seconds with both nostrils closed. If you are left-handed, place your left index and middle finger on your right nostril and inhale through the left before closing it with your thumb. After a few seconds, lift the thumb or fingers from the right nostril and exhale through it. Close the right nostril again, inhale through the left, and repeat the steps. Continue for 1–3 minutes. Over time, you may gradually increase the length of time for which you hold your breath, but never strain.

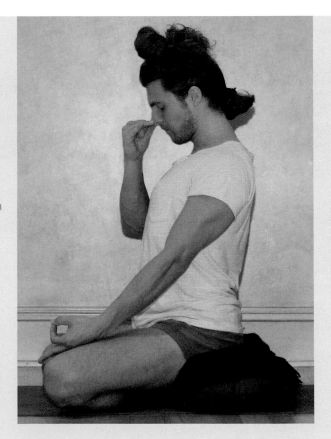

This pranayama is cooling to the body and mind. If you tend to be easily chilled, avoid doing it in winter. It is especially powerful to practice it under the light of the moon!

# Irritability

## FROM SNAPPY TO HAPPY

Feeling irritable can be characterized by feeling annoyed and frustrated, often over the little things in life. Irritability can become an all-consuming feeling of unease leading to cranky behavior, which tends to exacerbate an already uncomfortable situation. The root causes can be hormonal fluctuations—in men and women—stressful life events, insufficient sleep, and feelings of insecurity, fear, and sorrow, to name just a few. When grouchiness shows signs of becoming a consistent personality trait, it may need to be seriously addressed. Yoga can be an on-the-spot remedy for those times when your bad temper is situational, while a consistent practice of yoga can create a dynamic shift in perspective and help you bypass crankyland more often.

Do note, though, that it is entirely possible to feel irritated after yoga! Yoga practice is about traveling through the layers of the energy body, and as things shift, transform, open, and release, deeper feelings can surface. It's an exfoliation of the spirit, if you will. The good news is that usually if you come to yoga irritated, you leave in a better place, and if on occasion you don't, it's all part of a process that is still healthy and beneficial.

### 1. Salutations to the Sun (*Surya Namaskar A*)

Sun Salutations, sequences of poses, are described in full on pages 16–22. Sun Salutation A should flow quite quickly, so it's best to familiarize yourself with each pose first by practicing them all individually. If you think this sequence is too difficult or strenuous at this time, you may find Sun Salutation B more accessible.

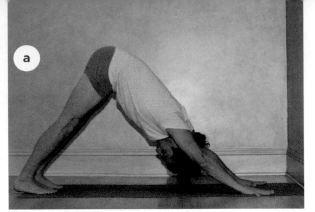

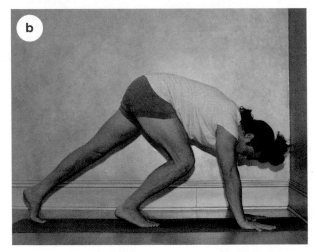

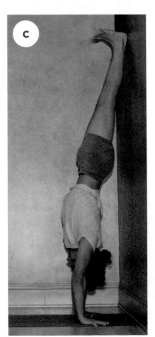

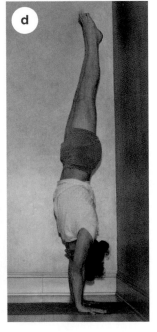

## 2. Handstand (*Adho Mukha Vrksasana*)

There's nothing like an inversion to shake things up and give you a new point of view! If you are brand new to handstand, try it first under the supervision of a professional teacher. If you are a beginner but have had some experience, a wall can serve you just fine. Please read through the instructions carefully before going upside down.

Start on hands and knees facing the wall with your hands 6–8 inches (15–20 centimeters) away from the wall. Come to Downward Dog (page 11) (**a**). Make sure you are breathing evenly, your body strong, your mind relaxed.

Step your dominant foot forward so that your knee lands more or less under your belly button. This leg is your spring (**b**). Push off and swing your other leg straight up to the wall with your bent leg following. Keep your arms straight! Either flex your feet as if you are standing on the ceiling (**c**) or push up through the balls of your feet. Look directly in front of you and keep your ears between your biceps.

If you wish to practice balancing, take one foot away from the wall and then the other, bringing your legs together strongly (**d**). You can look directly in front of you, or you might find that moving your focus point (*drishti*) toward the wall or your fingertips will help.

Stay up for as long as you feel comfortable, but remember to save enough strength and energy to come down. When you come down, bend at the hips, engage your belly and land either one or two feet at a time. Stand up slowly and see the world with fresh eyes. Repeat as desired.

**Variation:** L Pose is great for opening the shoulders and strengthening the upper body, and is a perfect choice if you are working up to handstand. Sit on the floor with your back against the wall and your legs stretched out in front of you. Note where your feet are, because this is where to place your hands.

Come to tabletop position facing away from the wall and place your hands on the spot where your feet were. Lift your hips into Downward Dog and bend your dominant leg so your foot is near your rear. Step that foot back onto the wall behind you. Lift your hips toward the sky as you bring your other leg up and straighten them both. It's likely your chest will be jutting out over your hands, so lift your hips higher, straighten your legs and move your chest toward the wall until your hands are under your shoulders or just a little way in front of them. Let your head hang between your arms with your gaze toward the wall (**above left**).

If you feel strong and can breathe easily, lift one leg at a time away from the wall for a few

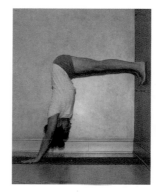
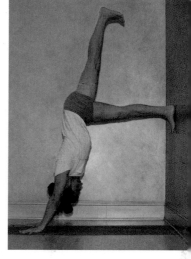

breaths (**above right**). This adds an element of strength and balance and prepares you for handstand.

The pose may feel very intense, and is not ideal for those with shoulder injuries. If neither Handstand nor L Pose work for you, stick with Downward Dog and hold for 3–10 breaths. Repeat as desired.

### 3. Reclining Butterfly (*Supta Baddha Konasana*)

Now that you have worked out some of the kinks, enjoy this tasty restorative pose, lying back over a bolster or folded blankets. Follow the instructions on pages 55–56 to get into the pose. Feel your breath, practice appreciation and forgiveness, and be present in this eternal now.

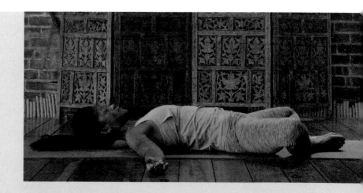

# Fear

## THE OTHER SIDE IS LOVE

In those moments when we are unable to embrace the unpredictable nature of life, fear can set in. There are many things to fear, but if we can master a few techniques, we have a better chance of feeling empowered to choose in which direction to go and where to put our focus. When the cold tingle of fear is creeping its way toward your heart, shift your attention to something or someone you love, breathe, and BE in that feeling. Keep it simple and keep it NOW. It is a good idea to warm up with 5 rounds of Sun Salutations A or B (pages 16–19) before beginning this section.

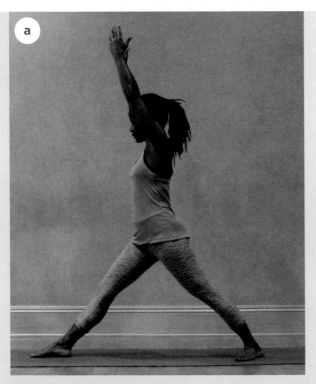

### 1. Warrior I (*Virabhadrasana 1*)

Start in *Tadasana* (page 9) and step or hop your feet wide apart (approximately 4 feet/ 1.25 meters). Stretch your arms out to your sides so that your wrists are above your ankles. Turn your left foot to the right at a 45 to 60-degree angle. Turn your right foot to the right at a 90-degree angle. Align your right heel with your left arch or heel. Turn your palms up, and lift your arms straight up, parallel with each other (**a**).

Turn your torso to the right, facing toward your right leg. Set a focus point (*drishti*). Inhale and reach through your fingertips, lengthening your spine.

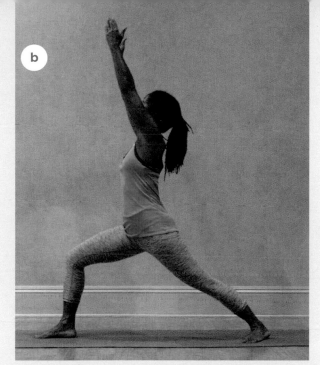

As you exhale, bend your right leg. Press strongly into your left heel and engage your core (**b**).

Align your biceps with your ears if possible, or let the arms open wider to accommodate tight shoulders. Stay for 3–5 breaths, then straighten the right leg. Repeat on the other side. Rest your hands on your hips to give your arms a break if needed.

**Variation:** When you lift your arms, face the palms forward and as you exhale through your mouth, bend the elbows and pull your hands down to either side of your ears with the palms still facing forward (**right**). This is a wonderful way to release tension in the heart center and activate the energy of courage that is seated in the heart chakra.

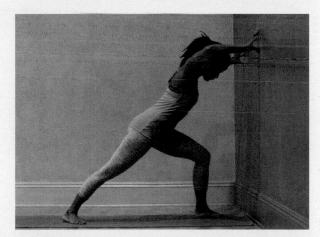

You can also step directly into Warrior I from Downward Dog (page 11) if you are practicing a vinyasa sequence.

**Modification:** You may find that this pose feels better with the support of a wall. Follow all the directions above from a few inches away from a wall, with your hands on your hips. Place your hands or fingertips on the wall when you bend your knee and lean slightly forward (**below right**).

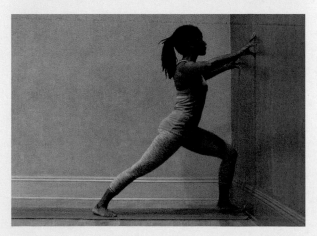

## 2. Warrior II (*Virabhadrasana II*)

From *Tadasana* (page 9) step your feet wide apart and extend your arms at shoulder height. Your ankles should line up under your wrists. Turn your left foot in on a 30-degree angle with your toes facing right. Turn your right foot out to face directly away from your body and pointing forward. Keep your spine upright, with your chest directly over your belly button and your hips square.

On an exhale, bend the right knee slowly while maintaining contact with the floor through the left heel. Make sure your right knee tracks over the second toe of your foot. Set your focus point (*drishti*) over the middle finger of your right hand. Relax your shoulders but keep the arms extended. Engage your abdominals and hold for 3–5 breaths. On an inhale, lift out of the pose and rest your hands on your hips. Turn your feet to the other side and repeat.

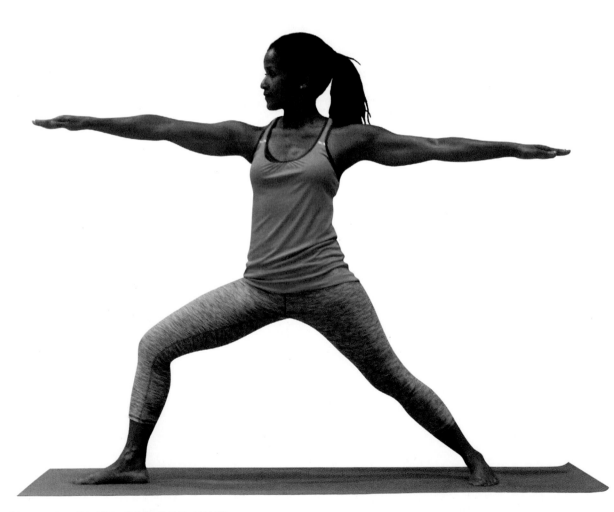

## 3. Camel Pose (*Ustrasana*)

Backbends open the heart center, which can build courage and release fear. Camel Pose is invigorating and uplifting, but it must be approached with care. If you are new to this pose, have a set of yoga blocks ready, one on the outside of each foot and on the highest level (see Modification, overleaf). If you have a back or neck injury, practice the Bridge instead (pages 60–61).

Start by kneeling upright on a mat or blanket, hips above knees and knees hip-width apart. You may have your toenails flat on the floor or tuck your toes under for a lift if you have a tender back. Place your hands on your hips and rotate your thighs inward a little so that your hip bones point forward rather than out to the sides.

Press firmly into the tops of your feet (or toes) and place your hands on your lower back with your fingers pointing down. Draw your shoulder blades into your back, opening the chest. Press the heels of your hands into your back and lengthen your sacrum. Feel the contrasting energy—rooting down into the legs and feet and lifting up through the chest and crown of the head (**a**).

Imagine you are lying back over a giant ball and begin to release your head back without dumping into your neck—keep it long. Breathe and notice how you feel. If you feel nervous or have trouble with your breath, back off a little for a couple of breaths. If you feel good, stay for 3–5 breaths (**b**).

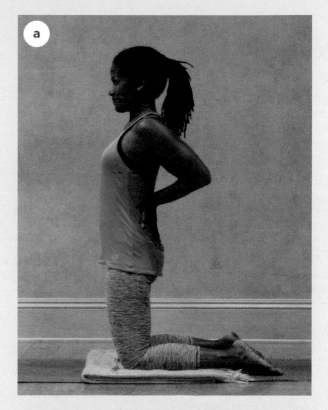

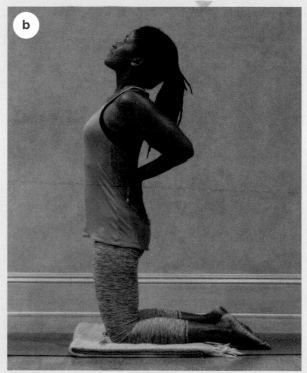

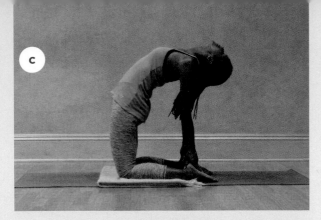

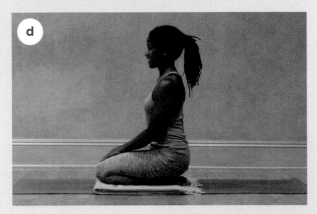

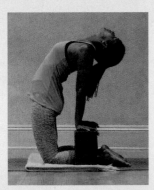

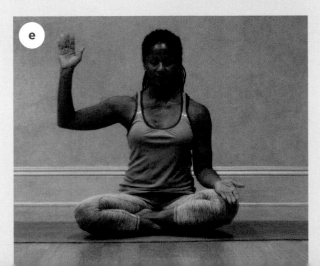

If you want to go deeper into the pose (you feel great and want more!), reach for your heels with your fingers pointing away from you. Once you have contact with your feet, lift up more through the chest, pulling your shoulder blades into your back and keeping the legs strong and hip points narrow. Look straight up toward the sky or gently release your head back, keeping length in the neck (**c**).

Hold for 3–5 breaths, then place your hands on your lower back, press down through your legs, and lift back up. Sit back on your heels with your ribs softened into your body (**d**).

Rest, breathe, feel. Repeat once or twice, resting in neutral between poses.

**Modification:** If your hands don't reach your feet, put your hands on blocks, one outside each ankle, fingers facing away from you. Adjust if needed so that the hands are directly under your shoulders (**left**).

When you have completed the asanas, you may wish to add a twist and, of course, rest in *Savasana* (page 13).

Before moving on with your day, spend a few extra moments (or even minutes) seated cross-legged in *Sukhasana* (page 10) or another comfortable position and take *Abhaya Mudra* (**e**). Bending at the elbow, lift your right hand to ear height, palm open, facing forward. Place your left hand face up on your left thigh or knee with the palm relaxed and open. Close your eyes and invite safety, reassurance, and divine protection into every cell in your body. This mudra represents peace, protection, and benevolence and dispels fear.

# Procrastination

## NO, NOW!

Even for those who are gifted at pulling through at the eleventh hour, procrastination has heavy repercussions on the body, mind, and spirit. I find that it is usually a by-product of wanting to exert control over a demanding life, albeit in a way that, as a habit, is not productive or healthy. It may be that it is connected to a task or duty we find distasteful, or something we must do that scares us. It may also be motivated by a lack of inspiration fueled by self-doubt. We will use poses that activate the solar plexus, our core chakra (*Manipura*), to empower and revitalize. Discipline is one of the key components to evolve in a yoga practice, and procrastination is its foil. Now let's get busy!

### 1. Plank (*Uttihita Chaturanga Dandasana*)

Plank packs a punch to the core muscles in the best way. It is an integral part of any vinyasa flow series, and is also used as a transition from standing to seated poses. You can come into the pose from Downward Dog (page 11) or from the floor.

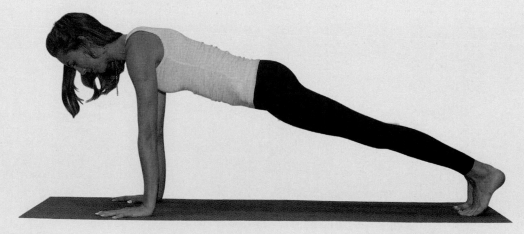

Starting from Downward Dog, you simply lift up onto the balls of your feet and roll your torso forward, like a wave, while pulling your belly button in toward your spine. Your hands may not line up under your wrists (where we want them), in which case you will need to shift a little to place them properly. The balls of your feet should be under your heels and hip-width apart. Soften your upper back so that it "melts" between your shoulder blades. Engage your abdominals and hug your triceps toward each other, keeping the shoulders moving away from your ears. The back of your head remains in line with your spine. Your body should slope gently from your shoulders to your hips to your heels, resembling a piece of wood that is on a slight incline.

To come into the pose from the floor, start in tabletop position with your hands under your shoulders and step one leg back at a time. Hold Plank for 3–5 breaths for 3 rounds. Rest either in Downward Dog (page 11) or Child's Pose (page 12) in between.

**Modifications:** If Plank is too much for your lower back, try Plank push-ups (**below left**).

Place your knees on the floor a few inches behind your hips and your hands under your shoulders. Tuck your toes under and cross your ankles. Lower your torso about 6 inches (15 centimeters), bending your elbows back behind you. Then push back up. Keep your abdominal muscles firm and your tailbone drawn into your body. Try not to round or puff up your upper back. Practice 5–10 push-ups for 1–3 rounds, inhaling as you lower and exhaling as you lift.

If you have shoulder or wrist injuries, try Dolphin Plank (**below right**). From tabletop position, place your forearms on the ground so that your elbows line up under your shoulders. Then step back one leg at a time. Keep your shoulders and hips on the same plane, your abdominal muscles firm, and remember to breathe! Hold for 3–10 breaths for 3 rounds and rest in between.

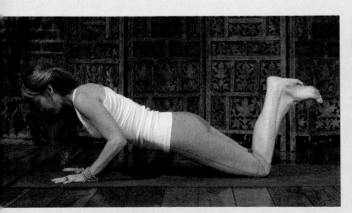

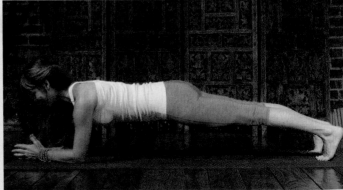

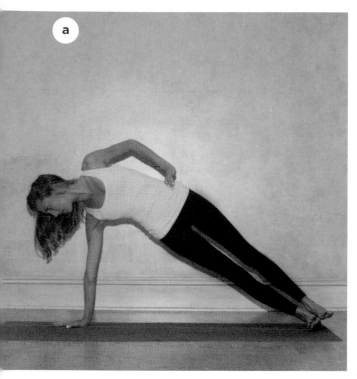

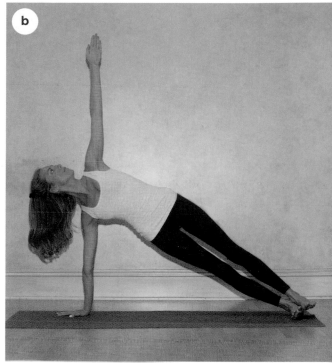

## 2. Side Plank (*Vasisthasana*)

*Vasistha* means "most excellent, best, and richest," and is the name of many great sages. This pose improves concentration and balance, and strengthens the arms, wrists, legs, and abdominals. While it is demanding, it embodies dynamic strength and optimism and can be a confidence booster.

Start in Downward Dog (page 11) and shift into Plank (pages 101–102). Move your hands a couple of inches in front of your shoulders. Roll to the outer right edge of your right foot and stack your left foot on top of the right. Place your left hand on your left hip. Be like a piece

of wood, firm and straight, and don't lift the hips high but keep them in that same incline as you had in Plank, only on its side. Both hip bones point straight ahead. Keep drawing the shoulder blades into your back and the abdominal muscles toward your spine (**a**).

You can extend your left arm straight up and turn your head to look at it (**b**), or keep the hand on the hip. Hold for 3–5 breaths on each side.

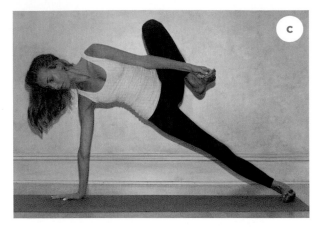

**Variation:** The variation here is actually a continuation into the full pose, but it is optional. Once you are established in the asana and feel safe and strong in your alignment, bend your left knee and reach for your left big toe, taking hold with yogi toelock (index and middle fingers together wrapped around the big toe) (**c**). Lift the leg up in the air directly above your left hip (**d**). Stay facing to the side as much as possible, drawing your tailbone into your body.

**Modifications:** This pose can be modified in three ways. The first is to set your right knee on the floor with your toes tucked and slightly out to the right of your body (**below left**).

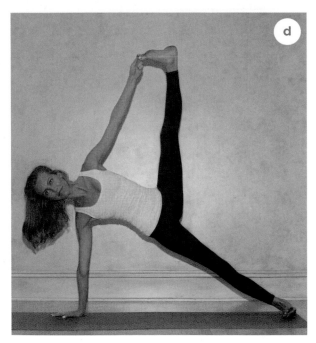

The second is to step your left leg in front of your right leg and place the foot flat on the floor under your left knee, facing forward in the direction of your hips (**below center**).

The third option is to place your right forearm on the floor with your elbow directly below your right shoulder and the fingers pointing forward in the direction of your hips (**below right**). Experiment to find the one that suits you best.

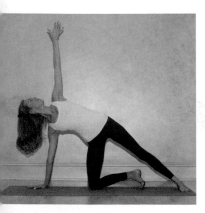

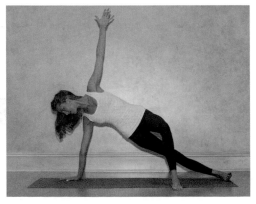

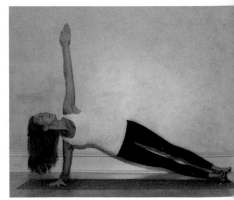

## 3. Both Feet (*Ubhaya Padangusthasana*)

The shape of this pose is, to me, an organic embodiment of the yogic journey toward light, bliss, *samadhi*. With the face and feet lifting in the same direction, reaching toward the sun like a flower, the feeling is noble and forthright yet humble. The excitement of holding the balance or risking a backward somersault is always exhilarating and comical. What better way to light a fire under your asana than to balance on the edge!

The pose can be realized in several ways. One is to begin in a seated forward fold, Intense Stretch of the West (pages 64–65). Sit on the floor with your legs straight out in front of you, spine straight, legs active, and feet flexed. Inhale as you stretch your arms straight up, and as you exhale, lower your hands toward your feet, extending your spine. Bend your knees and encircle the big toes with index and middle fingers together and the thumb in yogi toelock (**a**). Rock back on the sitting bones, firming the belly. Maintain a lift in the chest and extend the legs skyward. (**b**) It is important to keep the chest lifted and not allow the upper back to round, or you will find yourself flat on your back lickety split.

If you do end up rolling over, the second way to enter the pose is simply to come from another direction by continuing all the way back to Plow and, with the momentum of an inhale, engaging the core and rocking up to the sitting bones. Quickly tone the abdomen on an exhale (what I call belly brakes) and extend the legs.

A third way is to begin in Butterfly Pose (page 68), that is, sitting with spine straight and the soles of the feet together. Hold the big toes in yogi toelock, rock back with a lifted sternum, and stretch the legs up. Gaze steadily past the toes to help maintain balance. Once there, savor the pose for 30–60 seconds.

Both Feet is like a shot of hope to the nervous system, and once you are able truly to breathe in the pose, the steadiness (*stira*), joy, and ease (*sukha*) that are at the heart of the asana fill the yogi with a fragrance as delicious as the sweetest flower.

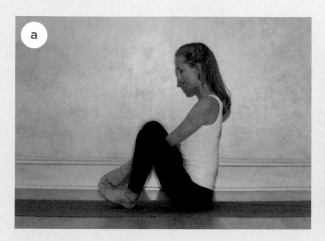

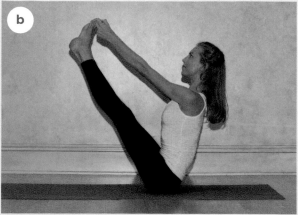

# Anger

## USE IT OR LOSE IT

Anger is a complex emotion. Yogis see it as existing halfway between the mental and physical plane, as all emotions do. When angry, we experience the release of adrenaline and noradrenaline into our nervous system. This is the match to the fuse of our feelings. Many emotions may be stacked up under anger—fear, sorrow, jealousy, injustice, to name a few. When properly channeled, anger can be the catalyst for positive change. However, it can also become a harmful reactive habit that is the result of a lack of tools to manage powerful feelings. While it might make you angry when someone says "chill out," it is precisely this mental cooling effect that yoga can give us, and it may just save the day. If you are someone who needs to move to release anger, start with Salutations to the Sun A or B (pages 16–19).

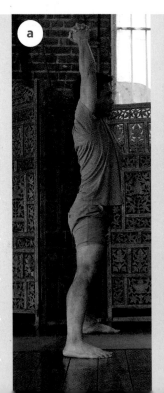
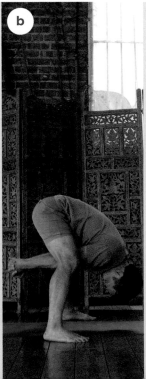

### 1. Straddle Pose or Expanded Feet Stretch (*Prasarita Padottanasana*) while chopping wood

One way to cool your jets is to release through sound and movement combined. I love this action because it's visceral and active. Begin standing straight in *Tadasana* (page 9). Put your hands on your hips and step your feet wide apart into Straddle Pose—the outer edges of your feet should be parallel and your heels aligned with each other. Stay there for a few breaths.

Then, keeping your legs in the pose, raise your arms over your head and clasp your hands, palms facing each other (**a**). Inhale with the arms up, and as you exhale bring the arms straight down and through your legs as you say "HAH!" (**b**). Keep your legs and abdominal muscles strong. Inhale and lift up again. Do this 3–5 times, then rest in a forward fold (page 11) or *Tadasana*. Repeat up to 3 times.

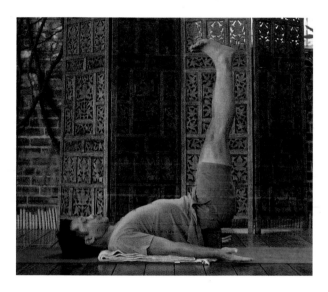

## 2. Shoulder Stand (*Salamba Sarvangasana*)

Follow the instructions on page 35 for Shoulder Stand—or if you have neck, wrist, or shoulder injuries, use a block and follow the instructions for Supported Shoulder Stand on pages 60–61 (**d**). This should feel good and not be difficult to hold. If it is, replace it with Legs up the Wall (page 30).

## 3. Lion's Breath (*Simhasana*)

You may feel silly and awkward as you get used to roaring like a lion, but a little silly can go a long way to soothe an angry beast. Also, this breath tones the throat and neck (even lions appreciate a youthful appearance), strengthens the platysma muscle at the front of the throat, releases jaw tension, and activates the bandhas. Choose your position: sit with big toes together and knees open, sit on your heels, or even lunge forward like a pouncing lion.

Take a big inhale, and as you forcefully exhale spread your hands like giant paws with claws,

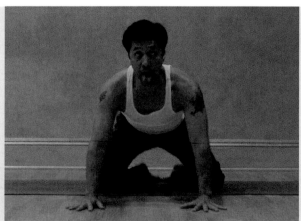

press them down into your legs or the floor, and simultaneously stick your tongue out and roll your wide-open eyes toward your third eye. Freeze for 20 seconds in the pose. Then relax and breathe normally. Repeat twice.

# Apathy

## WHY BOTHER?

Apathy can be the result of a creative or romantic dry spell, or erupt in the wake of overwhelming news or a series of challenging events. It can sneak up when the repetition of life and the existential question of the meaning of it all simply weigh the spirit down. By definition, apathy is a lack of emotion or feeling. The word emotion is derived from the Latin *emotere*, which means "energy in motion." Apathy isn't motivated enough even to be annoyed by its own listlessness, and is often characterized by lack of movement. However, yoga moves *prana*—life force, vitality, that which animates our being. *Prana* is physicalized in the breath and is the ideal antidote to apathy. The hard part is just getting going in the first place. If you are having a hard time, refer to Procrastination, page 101. Before starting the sequence, it would be a good idea to get your blood flowing with Salutations to the Sun A or B (pages 16–19).

### 1. One-legged King Pigeon (*Eka Pada Rajakapotasana*)

From Downward Dog (page 11), sweep your left leg up between your hands and lay it on the floor. Bend your left knee and try to make your leg parallel to the front edge of your mat if you are using one (**a**). Now follow the instructions (which also include variations and modifications) on pages 69–70 to move into the pose (**b**).

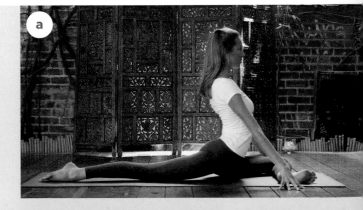

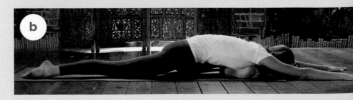

## 2. Half Moon (*Ardha Chandrasana*)

This pose is a hip and heart opening extravaganza. The strength and balance required pull the mind right into the body and therefore into the present. It activates the second (sacral) chakra (*Svadhisthana*), the seat of creativity and pleasure, and that's a boon for shifting out of an apathetic state of being. Have a block or books near the upper right corner of your mat if you are using one.

Start in *Tadasana* (page 9), place your hands on your hips, and step or jump the feet wide apart (approximately 4 feet/1.25 meters). Turn the left foot in 45 to 60 degrees and the right foot out 90 degrees. Extend your arms out to shoulder height with the palms facing down. Draw in your navel, lengthen your sacrum, and as you exhale bend the right knee to come into Warrior II (page 98). You can spend a couple of breaths enjoying Warrior II or head right into Half Moon.

Place your left hand on your left hip, inhale, and stretch your right side waist and right arm forward and toward the floor as you step your left foot up to the center of your mat. Shift your weight onto your right leg and lift your left leg up, with a firm thigh and flexed foot. If the floor is far from your right hand and you need to bend your knee a lot, grab your block or books and place your right hand on the support. In any case, align your right hand with your right shoulder.

Begin to straighten your right knee, being mindful not to lock or hyperextend it. Keep your ribs drawing into your body, your left leg

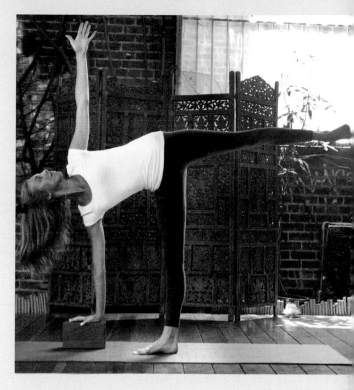

active, and, if you feel stable, lift your left arm to the sky. Turn your head to gaze at your left thumb, which should line up with your nose. Your inner left foot is parallel with the floor. Check to see that your right foot is pointing straight ahead and the knee is lined up over your shin bone for maximum hip rotation. Stay for 3–5 breaths and enjoy the subtle yet powerful luminosity of moon energy as it brings you to life. Repeat on the other side.

**Variation:** Follow the instructions for Half Moon; then bend the leg that is in the air and grab your foot with your hand. Keep your core strong and open your shoulder gently and with breath for a deeper heart, hip, and mind opener. This is *Ardha Chandra Chapasana*.

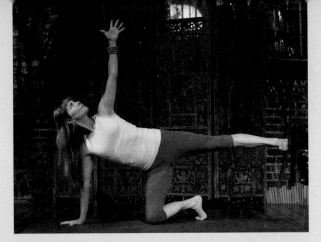

knee. Your right hand is underneath your right shoulder. Press your left foot flat on the floor on a 45 to 60-degree angle. Your left hand is on your hip. When you feel stable, lift your left leg to hip height and flex the foot. Then lift your left arm up and gaze at your thumb. You have created a mini moon!

Another alternative is to follow the instructions for Half Moon but position yourself a few inches from a wall for added support. This is a good choice if you are pregnant.

**Modifications:** If this pose is out of reach at the moment, come to tabletop position and shift your weight to your right knee, moving your right toes a few inches to the right of your

### 3. Sun Breath (*Surya Bhedana*) with Life Force Mudra (*Prana Mudra*)

We have harnessed the inspiration of the moon, so now we will invoke the energy of the sun for a balanced remedy that is sure to inspire. Sit in a comfortable seat and with the left hand touch the pads of the thumb, ring finger, and pinky together, extending the index and middle fingers for *Prana Mudra*. This is the mudra of vitality and life energy.

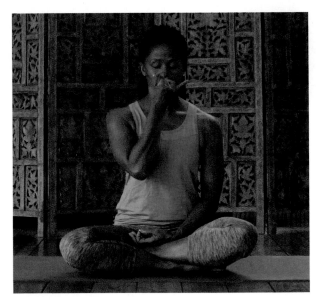

Now place the right hand into Deer Seal (*Mrigi Mudra*) by pressing the middle and index fingers firmly into the palm and slipping the pinky fingernail underneath the pad of the ring finger. If this is difficult, switch to *Vishnu Mudra* by leaving the pinky finger free (**right**). You can switch hands if you are a lefty. Place the ring finger onto the left nostril, inhaling through the right. Gently pinch both nostrils shut, using the thumb on the right nostril, then lift the fingers

and exhale through the left. Continue so that you always inhale through the right and exhale through the left, for 1–3 minutes. This breath can cultivate perseverance, enthusiasm, and zeal, and renew your hope. When finished, meditate, then congratulate yourself on taking a powerful step in the right direction.

# Depleted and Overwhelmed

## WHEN THE WIND HAS LEFT YOUR SAILS

When we feel drained, it may feel as if fog has settled on the horizon and it's not possible to imagine the sun shining simply because it takes too much energy or vision to do so. It is known that intense and chronic stress can produce or exacerbate adrenal fatigue, fibromyalgia, hormone depletion, immune disorders, and other health concerns. However, if we are tuning in to ourselves, we may catch the signs and symptoms before we are overwhelmed. Recognizing when you need to recharge, and working a little breather into your life as a priority, can be the "apple a day that keeps the doctor away."

### 1. Sweet Pose (*Sukhasana with a Chair*) and Victorious Breath (*Ujjayi Pranayama*)

Sit cross-legged on the floor in front of a chair, spine straight, in *Sukhasana* (page 10). If your low back feels tight, sit up on a folded blanket or two. You may also place a blanket or towel on the seat of the chair for extra comfort. Cross your forearms and place your forehead on your arms. Relax into the pose.

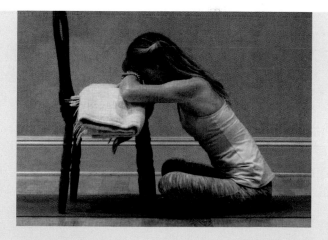

This requires little to no physical effort and should feel very comfortable. Focus on your breathing. Notice it and draw your attention away from everything else. Feel your breath moving in your body. Tune your awareness to, and lightly constrict, your throat before inhaling through your nose. Feel the sensation and listen for the sound of your own breath like a "whoosh" or ocean waves. Exhale in the same manner, listening for that sound (*Ujjayi Pranayama*, pages 28-29). If you are having trouble hearing it, exhale through an open mouth. Then close your mouth and try again.

Listen to the ocean in your body, until you feel calm and connected to the breath and this moment. You may desire to keep your attention on the breath or release into a soft, natural breath, allowing yourself to move into a state of *pratyahara*—withdrawal of the senses. Stay here as long as you are comfortable.

**Modifications:** Rather than sitting cross-legged, you can stretch your legs out in front of you or place them in a V if that feels more comfortable. If they are straight out, they will slide under the chair seat. If they are in a V, they will go around the outside of the chair legs.

## 2. Supported Child's Pose (*Salamba Balasana*)

For this cozy, restorative pose you will need a bolster and/or several folded blankets. Begin on hands and knees and bring your big toes together, knees apart. Sit back on your heels and draw your navel toward your spine. Pull the support in between your knees up to your groin or abdomen and lean forward so that your torso and head are lying along the prop. Send your hips toward your heels. Stay for as long as you are comfortable, with a minimum of 5 minutes, turning your head to one side and then the other for an equal length of time.

**Modifications:** If you have any discomfort in your ankles, place a blanket beneath your feet. If your knees or quadriceps are tight, place a blanket or something similar evenly and snugly behind your knees before taking your hips back.

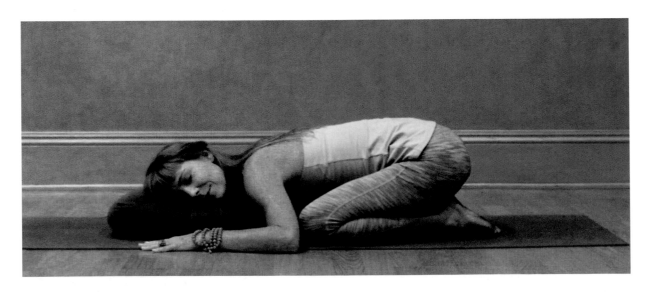

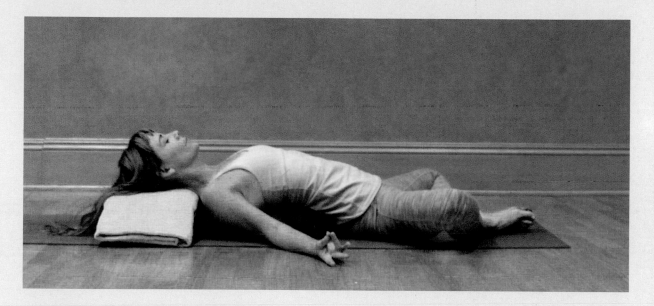

### 3. Reclining Butterfly (*Supta Baddha Konasana*) with yogic breathing

Follow the instructions on pages 55–56 to get into the pose.

Now practice *Dirga* or *Ujjayi* breathing. For *Dirga* breath, inhale into the bottom of your belly, then your solar plexus, and finish in your chest. Pause briefly and then exhale from the upper chest, solar plexus, and finally bottom of the belly.

For *Ujjayi* breathing, inhale through your nose while tuning your awareness to, and lightly constricting, your throat. Feel the sensation and listen for the sound of your own breath like a "whoosh" or ocean waves. Exhale in the same manner.

Once you feel settled and focused again, go back to taking easy, natural breaths and visualize yourself floating in water. By releasing tension in the hips and gently stretching the abdomen, this pose restores harmony to the second (sacral) chakra (*Svadhisthana*), which is governed by water. It activates and restores our senses of power and comfort, easing anxiety and pacifying an irritable mind. Stay for as long as you like.

**Variation:** If you prefer, you can lie with your legs up the wall (page 30) while practicing yogic breathing.

If you are going to meditate after practicing these asanas, which I strongly recommend, take *Prithvi Mudra* by bringing the thumb and ring finger of each hand to touch (**above**). This mudra decreases the element of fire energy and increases the earth (*kapha*) element, which helps to restore, rebuild, and prevent burnout. It is a replenishing mudra.

# Obsessive

## LET GO AND LET GO AGAIN!

In more and more studies, yoga is shown to have powerful effects on the obsessive personality, be it in behavioral tendencies or physiological mental disorder. It may be your go-to "medicine" or an effective supplement to your current protocol, but practiced with consistency, yoga can reflect back to you your true and perfect nature and bring some light and relief. If you have the time, practice the morning, noon, or night sequence (pages 160–73), according to the time of day, before the following poses. You should definitely warm up with one of these sequences if you are going to practice the first posture, Bow Pose. If you don't have the time for that, skip Bow Pose and start with the chant. Then proceed to Moon Breath and *Shanmukhi Mudra*, finishing in *Savasana* (page 13). Try to practice this sequence of pranayama, mudra, and meditation daily if you are in a particularly difficult state of mind.

### 1. Bow Pose (*Dhanurasana*)

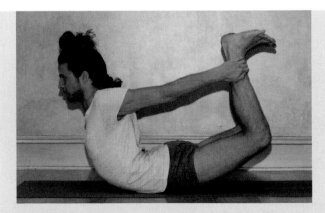

Come onto your belly and place your forehead on the floor. Bend your knees and reach back for your ankles or the tops of your feet. Wrap the thighs in toward each other, roll your shoulder blades in, and lift the heads of the shoulders off the floor. When you inhale, push back with your legs and lift your body up so that only your pelvis and lower abdomen remain on the floor. Gaze forward, or lengthen your neck and take your head back, being careful not to compress the back of the neck too much. Stay here as long as your breath comes evenly, then rest on your belly with your head on your hands.

## 2. Chant: The Seven *Bijas* Mantra

*Bijas* are the seed sounds of the seven major energy centers (chakras) in the body. Chakra means "wheel of light" in Sanskrit, and each one is an energy vortex, which both receives and radiates energetic vibration. Each chakra corresponds to particular aspects of mental and physical health. When we chant, the sounds we activate balance and purify the chakra with sound vibration.

In Sanskrit, "*man*" means "to think" and "*tra*" means "tools or instruments." So mantras are repetitious, energetically charged, vibrational tools of thought. When we focus on these one-syllable seed sounds, we can disrupt patterns of thought that are not serving us, while at the same time creating a more positive and balanced vibration in the body.

Sit comfortably and place your hands in any mudra or position that feels good to you. You can chant the seven *bijas* in order from lowest to highest in the body one at a time, or you can chant one *bija* as many times as you like before moving on. The *bijas* are:

**1—LAM**  root chakra (pelvic floor and perineum) (*Muladhara*)

**2—VAM**  sacral chakra (2 inches/5 centimeters below the belly button to the pelvic floor) (*Svadhisthana*)

**3—RAM**  solar plexus chakra (*Manipura*)

**4—YAM**  heart center chakra (*Anahata*)

**5—HAM**  throat chakra (*Vishuddha*)

**6—OM**  third eye chakra (*Ajna*)

**7—Silence or OM**  crown chakra (crown of the head) (*Sahasrara*)

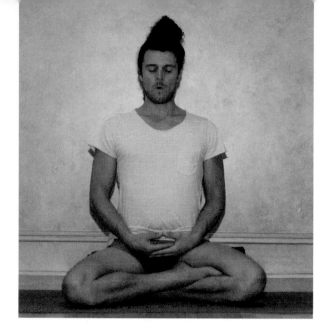

There are two pronunciations for the first six *bijas*. They can be pronounced with a long A ("ahhh") and sound like "long" or a "U" sound as in "yum". See which resonates with you. *Om* is pronounced with a long O ("ohhh"). Try to balance out the length between the middle and end of the sound—that is, extend the "mmm" as close to the "ahhh" or "ohhh" sound as possible—which gives a more potent vibration. (This is a little different from the way you may be used to chanting *Om* before a class, when we tend to keep the middle "ohhh" sound long and shorten the "mmm" sound at the end. See also page 159.)

Chant for 3–5 minutes, then rest in *Savasana* (page 13).

**Modification:** Although it is ideal to sit with a straight spine for the purposes of allowing the prana to flow upward, you may lie on your back if you are especially tired or simply feel more at ease that way.

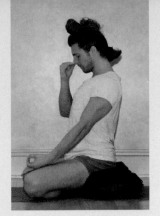

### 3. Moon Breath (*Chandra Bhedana*)

Follow the instructions on page 92 for Left Nostril Breathing.

### 4. Closing the Seven Gates (*Shanmukhi Mudra*)

This mudra is quite powerful and guides us toward a state of *pratyahara* (withdrawal of the senses) by sealing the ears, eyes, nose, and mouth, decreasing our sensitivity to stimuli. While distracting ourselves with external stimuli can be effective in decreasing obsessive thought patterns, a practice of *pratyahara* is soothing to the nerves and fosters ease in the body, which translates to the agitated mind.

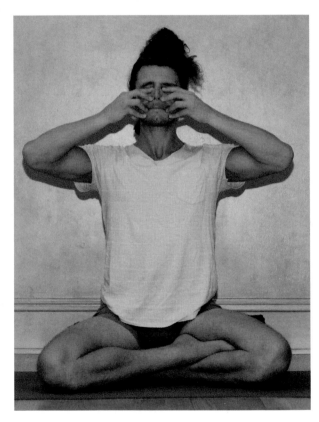

Take a comfortable seated position with your spine straight. Lift your arms and elbows so that you are able to close your ears with your thumbs, your eyes gently (not pressing the cornea) with your index fingers, and your nostrils with your middle fingers. Place your ring fingers above your mouth, and your pinky fingers below your mouth.

Lift your middle fingers from your nostrils and inhale slowly. Close your nostrils and retain the breath for a comfortable length of time before lifting your fingers and exhaling through your nose. This is one round. If you are new to pranayama practices, practice 5–10 rounds. For those who have more experience (especially with alternate nostril breathing, page 89), work toward 5–10 minutes and rest as needed.

When you remove your hands from your face and open your eyes, you may find that your vision is slightly blurred. Relax and wait—your eyes will soon readjust and feel refreshed.

# The Blues

## PRETTY COLOR—UGLY FEELING

While the beautiful blues of the ocean and sky may evoke feelings of spaciousness and appreciation for vast natural beauty, as an emotional state blue is a horse of a different color. Falling somewhere between sorrow and apathy and shuffling on the edge of depression, the blues may be excellent fodder for some of our favorite pieces of music and art, but the reality of being in a blue rut is nowhere near as romantic as it may sound.

### 1. Tree Pose (*Vrksasana*) with Lotus Mudra

Balances are always effective for pulling us out of the past (where many of the blues take seed) and into the NOW.

Follow the instructions for Tree Pose on pages 84–85, but instead of adopting *Hakini Mudra*, add Lotus Mudra. The meaning of mudra is "delight or pleasure" (*mud*) and "to draw forth" (*ra*), so we will extract something delightful from the rubble. This happens to be the symbolism of the lotus flower. It grows in the murky, dense goo at the bottom of the lake or river and moves unerringly toward the light for a year before bursting to the surface in all its resonance and glory, unstained by its grimy beginnings. During the time it blooms, the flower closes at night and submerges itself below the surface of the water, rising to the surface again the next day with the sun.

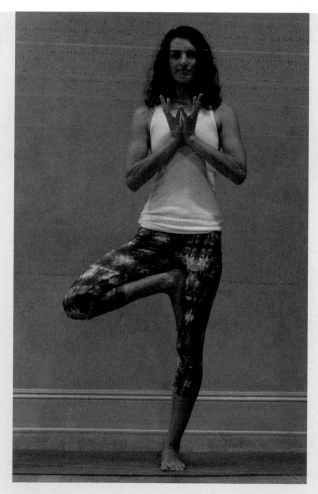

Contained in its seed are tiny leaves that are the exact miniature of the full-grown flower. We make this journey from dark to light countless times in our lives. The trick is in blooming to the light of the new day without carrying the stains of the past with us.

Place the heels of your hands, the pinkies, and the thumbs to touch and spread the rest of the fingers open wide. Place the mudra at heart center once you are steady in Tree Pose. You may enjoy lifting the mudra up to the sky for a few breaths and imagining the healing vibrancy of life-giving sun pouring into your veins. Feel yourself reawaken to the present and all the wonder that your future holds.

## 2. Handstand, Headstand, L Pose, or Downward Dog

Basically, pick an inversion, because getting your feet over your head will shake things up in all the right ways! Choose from Handstand (**right** and page 94), Headstand (**far right** and pages 86–87), L Pose (**below** and page 95), and Downward Dog (**below right** and page 11).

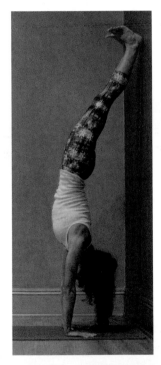

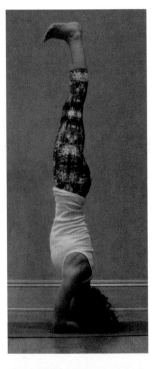

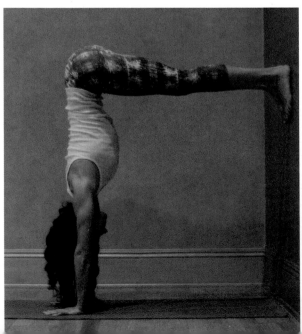

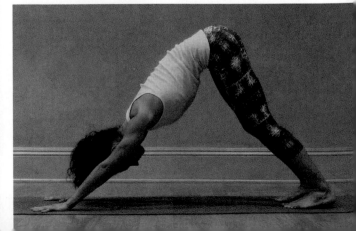

### 3. Skull Shining Breath (*Kapalabhati*) with bandhas

Sit cross-legged on the floor, or on a chair with your feet flat on the ground. Bring your hands into *Jnana Mudra* with the thumb and index fingers touching to form a circle and the arms extended. Inhale fully through your nose and exhale through your mouth. On your next inhale, stop short of a full breath and exhale through your nose with a forceful blow as your abdomen engages toward your navel. Let your inhale follow naturally. The focus in this practice is on the exhale, which comes from the action of the belly pulling in. The inhale is slow in a natural reaction to the force of the exhale. Both breaths are done through the nose.

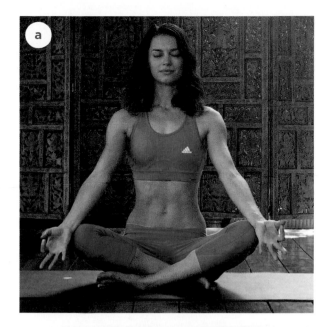

Now let's add something extra to uplift you even more. Lift the arms straight up in the air and then open them to form a wide V. Fold all your fingers but not your thumbs into your hands and point your thumbs toward each other and slightly down. If it's more comfortable for your shoulders, bend your elbows a little.

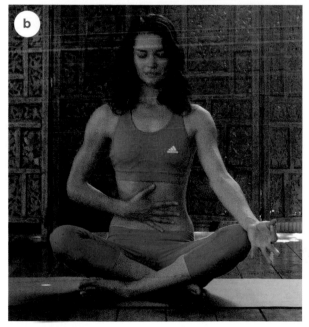

Begin your skull shining breath. When you finish your first round, empty all the breath out. Then inhale with your arms still up, and as you exhale through your mouth, bring the arms straight down and your hands into *Jnana Mudra*—palms up with the thumb and index fingertips together—on your legs (**a**). Holding the exhale, squeeze your pelvic floor (*Mula Bandha*), engage your abdominals and lift them up (*Uddiyana Bandha*), inhale a sip of air and bow the chin to the chest (*Jalandhara Bandha*) (**b**). Hold as long as you are comfortable and then release *Mula Bandha* and *Uddiyana Bandha*, and as you release *Jalandhara Bandha* inhale the rest of the breath before letting it all go with an exhale through your mouth.

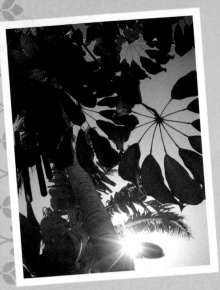

# PART 3

# Remedies for the Spirit

WHEN YOU KNOW WHAT YOU WANT,
OR WANT ANOTHER HELPING OF WHAT
YOU HAVE!

### Spirit

"The principle of conscious life; the vital principle in humans,
animating the body or mediating between body and soul"

### Soul

"The spiritual part of humans as distinct from the physical
part; the emotional part of human nature; the seat of the
feelings or sentiments"

### Nourish

"To sustain with food or nutriment; supply with what is
necessary for life, health, and growth; to cherish, foster, keep
alive, etc."

The spirit is like air—utterly invisible to the naked eye and yet essential
and intrinsic to all of life. The spirit is the spark that leads to the bonfire
of experience. It is the genesis, the lightbulb, the godseed within. When
we are in touch, connected, and communicating with ourselves, we are
speaking the language of the soul, and all that is sacred and special is
in our awareness. To feed the spirit, to nourish our inner life and find
its tangibility, the way we know we are breathing air, and must breathe
air to live, is to shift from a life of repetition and confusion to a life of
purpose and meaning, and maintain that for a lifetime.

It is easy to believe in only what we can see or physically feel. The body is right there, made of blood, flesh, and bone. We know when we are hurt because there is visible evidence. We know when we are hungry because the belly literally growls to be fed. We know when we are sick because the body slows and weakens. The spirit speaks in a language no less dynamic, but one that requires a deft ear and willing mind to translate. The universe comprises a multitude of invisible forces that affect our daily lives. There's atmospheric pressure, ozone layers, shifts in light and sound waves, and so on and on. An antonym for "animated" is "spiritless." If we don't pay attention to our deepest longings, callings, and desires, we have no animation, no spirit. Our interior landscape would be like a black hole, potential yet untapped.

*Prana*, Sanskrit for "original life force," breaks down to "*pra*," which is constant, and "*an*," which is movement. This energetic life force is in constant motion, and the practice of pranayama uses the life force of breath to move our energy in an organized fashion and with focus. Swami Satyananda Saraswati explains, "Modern physiology describes two types of nervous systems, the sympathetic and the parasympathetic, and these two nervous systems are interconnected in each and every organ of the body. In the same way, every organ is supplied with the energy of prana and the energy of mind."

My life has led me to see this as the spirit/soul of humans being the creative team, the life force in action, and the mind/consciousness being the grand organizer, ensuring that we bring out our potential and make it manifest in the world. This potential may be to live a life of kindness, to cure disease, or to find harmony within our own being. It is up to each individual to learn the language and message of his or her own spirit, and it is the magic of the life journey to do so.

We will use the practice of yoga to connect with, to listen to, and even to request a higher awareness of what it is that animates us and brings our heartsong to life.

*"I have been a seeker and I still am, but I stopped asking the books and the stars. I started listening to the teaching of my Soul."*
Rumi

# Love

## IT REALLY IS WHERE IT'S AT

When we turn our attention to love in any form, it shifts our immediate experience. Focusing on what and whom we love can color our perceptions of the day, or even our lives, almost instantaneously. The heart, which is the energetic center for the feeling of love, is remarkably resilient and tenacious both physically and emotionally. The desire to give and receive love is as mighty as this muscular organ's ability continuously to pump between 1,500 and 2,000 gallons of blood per day through the body. Love is at the core of our reason for being in the way that the sun is the center of the solar system. It is around this that all becomes, and all revolves. Let's get our love on.

### 1. The Remover of Obstacles (*Ganesha Mudra*)

Since love is our true nature, the only reason for experiencing a dearth of that lovin' feeling is that something is in the way—an obstacle impeding the flow of love toward ourselves and others. A feeling, memory, or perception has us stuck in the past or fearful of the future, like a boulder on our path. If we address the physical center of love (the heart center), we can get some leverage to move that rock, or find a way around it, and wipe away the illusion that we are separated from love.

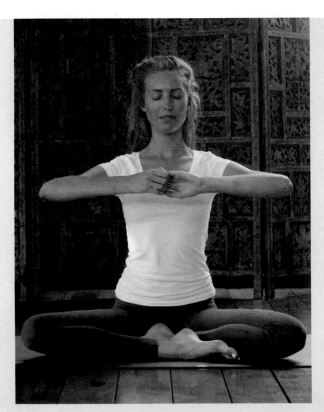

Sit comfortably cross-legged in *Sukhasana* or *Siddhasana* (page 10), raise your arms to chest height, and hook the fingers of one hand over the fingers of the other, elbows bent out to the sides. Inhale, feeling the chest expand and the heart chakra (*Anahata*) ignite. As you exhale, pull strongly on your gripped fingers but don't release them. This will stimulate the meridian lines and pranic flow in the region of the heart. Do this 3 times, then rest for one natural breath and repeat with the other hand in front. Take a few moments to be with your sensations before moving on.

## 2. Chant: *Lokah Samastah Sukhino Bhavantu*

In the same way that singing can be an elixir for the spirit, chanting can be a vibrational game changer. You don't need to be a singer or even be able to carry a tune. Simply let the sound pour out from the heart in whatever way you find comfortable. It may be quiet or loud, fast or slow. Most important, when using Sanskrit, is simply to have the correct pronunciation. Sanskrit chanting has a powerful effect on the nervous system. It is documented to enhance brainwave activity, release the healing agent melatonin (owing to the placement of the tongue on particular meridians in the mouth), lower the levels of stress hormones released into the body, and purify and cleanse the energy body. Sound has a clear effect on animals, humans, and even plants, and when we take it a step farther and chant with a specific intention and pattern, it becomes a transformational remedy.

With this chant we are invoking "*ahimsa*," which is the practice of non-violence, which is central to yoga. When we practice *ahimsa* toward ourselves and others, we are motivated

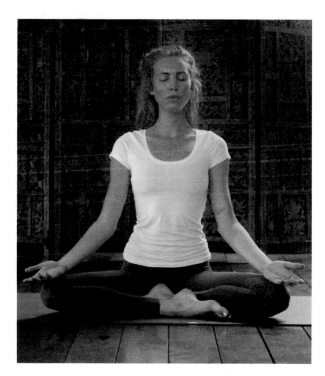

by compassion and love. The words "*lokah samastah sukhino bhavantu*" (pronounced "low-kaw saahh-maahh-staahh soo-kee-no baahh-vaahhnn-too") mean: "May all beings everywhere be happy and free and may the thoughts, words, and actions of my own life contribute in some way to that happiness and to that freedom for all."

Chant these Sanskrit words for 1–3 minutes or as long as you like.

### 3. Supported Fish (*Salamba Matsyasana*) with guided meditation

Follow the instructions on page 36 to come into Supported Fish pose. If you can do so while pressing your feet against a wall, so much the better, but it's not essential. The aim is to have an earthy, grounded feeling so that you feel safe and supported to open through the heart center. Visualize the way a fish leaps out of the water and allow that freedom and lightness to come into your chest as you stay anchored through your legs.

Once you are comfortably in the pose, close your eyes and turn your attention to your breath. Feel it coming into your heart center and visualize a flower bud there, perhaps a lotus flower or any that you love. With each gentle inhale, see the petals begin to open. With each exhale, relax into the slow unfolding of the flower.

Continue with this visualization until the flower is fully bloomed in the center of your chest. Then inhale in three parts, or "sniffs," drawing in the sweetness of the moment, and exhale all tension from body and mind through an open mouth. Do this 3 times, then rest and breathe naturally.

Leave the pose when you are ready, easing onto one side, bending your knees, and rolling up to a seated position or pushing down with your hands and sitting up with bent knees. Take a few moments to feel the effects of your renewed and open heart.

**Variation:** Once you are in Supported Fish, you can leave your legs stretched straight out or, for an added hip opener that is especially delicious, bring the soles of the feet together in Butterfly Pose (**below**). If the hips feel a bit tight, add a block or a book under each knee.

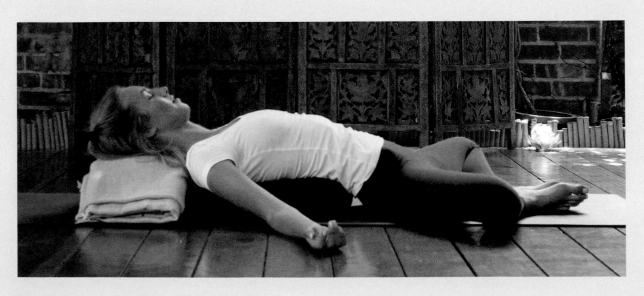

# Joy

## CAPTURE THE RAPTURE

Joy has a mystical, spiritual quality that resonates more profoundly than happiness. Happiness, while tasty, is centered on the "I" and can feel fleeting, leaving us hungry for more, while joy expands our attention and our awareness beyond ourselves and connects us in a primal way to feeling and being a part of all that is. The physical center for joy is the solar plexus. Connecting to your core by strengthening and stretching can activate feelings of confidence and worthiness, and therefore nurture your capacity for joy. When you are centered from within and accepting of yourself, you can more easily access joy and have your "fun in the sun." Warm up with a few rounds of Sun Salutations (pages 16–22) before beginning the following sequence.

### 1. Boat Pose (*Navasana*) with Mudra for Happiness

What better way to evoke your own sunny nature than on a boat! From a sitting position, bend your knees and place your feet on the floor. Rock back, supporting yourself with your hands, and point your feet so that just your toes touch the floor. Lift your feet off the floor, keeping your knees bent, then extend your feet so that they are at the same height as your knees. Point your toes, or flex the balls of your feet and fan your toes. Lift and extend your arms to either side of your legs, engaging your abdominal muscles. Keep your spine straight and your chest lifted (**a**).

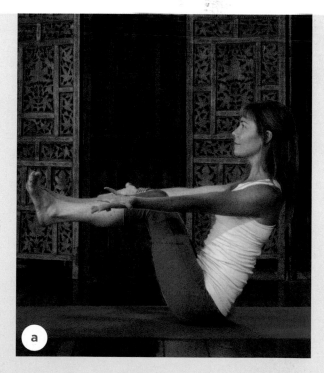

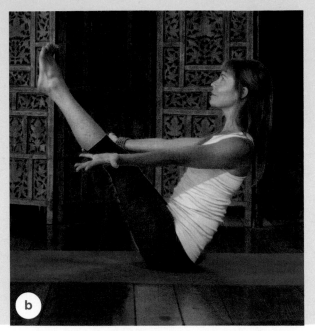

**b**

If you feel good here, continue to extend your legs to straight (**b**). If you have back pain, or it is too difficult for any reason, bend the knees again. You may also feel better clasping your hands behind your knees. Take 3–5 breaths, then come down, cross your legs, and, sitting tall, take the Mudra for Happiness by lifting the arms to shoulder height, bending the elbows, and making peace-sign fingers. Hold the ring and pinky fingers in with your thumb. Take 3–5 breaths and then return to the Boat one more time, finishing with the Mudra for Happiness, holding it for 1–3 minutes.

## 2. Upward Facing Bow
### (*Urdhva Dhanurasana*)

Known "on the street" as Wheel Pose, this deep backbend could be called a "joystick" it's so mood-enhancing. You may remember it from happy gymnastic days as a child.

Lie on your back with your feet flat on the floor under your knees and parallel to each other. Bend your elbows and place your hands alongside your ears a few inches away from your head, palms down and fingers pointing toward your feet (**a**). As you inhale, push yourself up onto the top of your head by pressing evenly into hands and feet. Pause briefly to pull your shoulder blades into your back and down away from your ears (**b**). Then, on your next inhale, push up to the full pose by pressing firmly into all four corners of your feet and your wide outstretched hands. Keep your

knees over your ankles and the feet pointing straight ahead (**c**). Breathe!

When you are ready to release, tuck your chin into your chest and slowly lower down, with your head moving slightly toward your fingertips. Rest on your back with the soles of your feet together and your knees open in Reclining Butterfly, or with the feet on the floor hip-width apart or wider and the knees dropping in to touch. Repeat if desired.

Finish with either of these twists. Draw your knees in to your chest and, as you exhale, gently drop them both to one side with the feet stacked on top of each other. Stretch your arms out wide at shoulder height, and roll your head away from your legs. Alternatively, draw your right knee in to your chest, keeping the other leg extended on the floor. On an exhale, draw your right leg across your body with your left hand. Stretch the right arm out at shoulder height and roll your head toward the

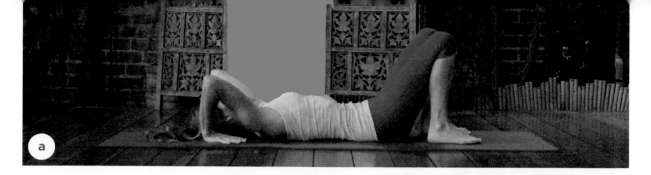

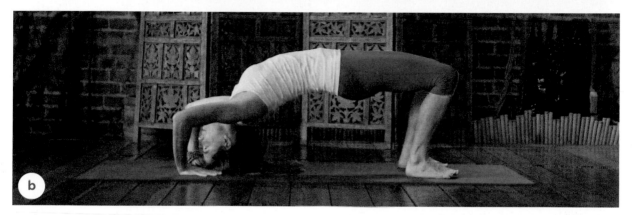

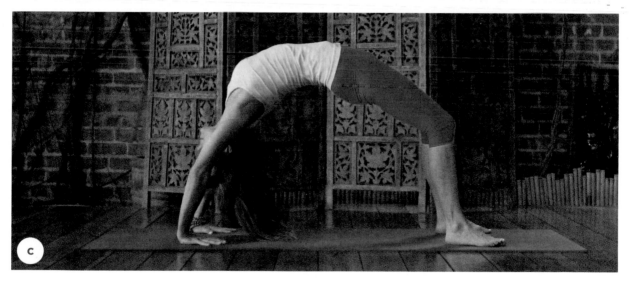

outstretched arm. Whichever one you choose, after 3–5 breaths repeat on the other side.

**Modification:** For a less strenuous but still joyful backbend, practice Bridge Pose (page 60).

Rest in Reclining Butterfly in between Bridges by lying on your back with the soles of the feet together, one hand on your heart and one hand on your belly. When you are finished, hug the knees to the chest and make slow circles with them to massage the low back.

# Peace

## COMING SOON TO A BODY NEAR YOU

To catch a ride on the peace train, we need to employ the understanding that it is not external events or situations that dictate our inner state of being—although life can throw us many a major doozy, for sure. Rather, our inner reality affects our perception of the outer reality. When we use the yogic tools of asana, pranayama, and meditation, we can mute knee-jerk reactions that often arise out of fear, stay in the moment, and actively practice peace. Being peaceful is a choice and an action, although it looks and feels like stillness.

### 1. *Shanti Mudra* (Invocation of Peace)

Sit cross-legged in *Sukhasana* or *Siddhasana* (page 10) and take *Bhairava Mudra* or *Bhairavi Mudra*. *Bhairava Mudra* is practiced by placing the right hand in the palm of the left hand (which is the masculine aspect), both facing up (**a**). *Bhairavi* is done with the left hand in the palm of the right hand (which is the feminine aspect), both facing up. You can do either or both, according to the aspect you want to increase.

Relax the body and exhale completely. Hold the breath out and engage root lock (*Mula Bandha*) by squeezing the perineum, which will feel as if you are slightly lifting the pelvic floor, or like a Kegel exercise. Hold for as long as you can without straining. When you release, begin to inhale, and with the palms facing

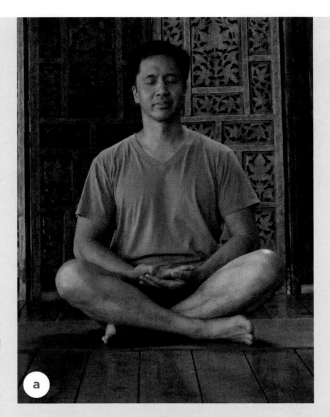

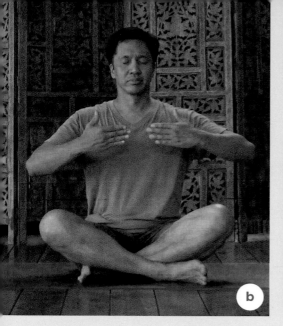
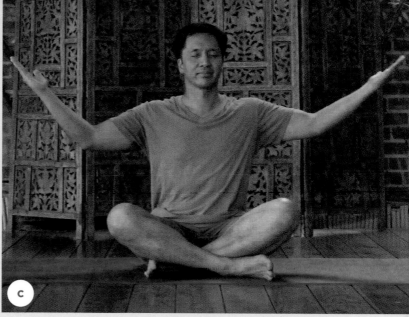

your body and a few inches away, the fingers close but not touching, move the hands slowly up until they are in front of your throat. Your arms and hands should be soft and floaty and your elbows bent out to the side (**b**). Once you have reached your maximum inhalation, hold the breath and stretch your arms out to the sides, palms facing up, with soft elbows (**c**). Keep everything relaxed. Stay as long as you comfortably can and then reverse the directions of the hands as you exhale, finishing

in the mudra. Rest for a few breaths and repeat 3–7 times.

Feel the life force (*prana*) moving up the body with the hands, swelling and spreading ease and peace into every cell and lighting up each of the seven chakras as your hands move along. When your arms open, radiate peace and wellbeing to the universe. On the way down, with your exhale, imagine the *prana* moving down your spine and anchoring you safely and firmly to the earth.

### 2. Butterfly Pose (*Baddha Konasana*)

Follow the instructions on page 68 to come into Butterfly Pose. In the restorative version of the pose shown here, place your hands on your calves and a block between your feet, then lean forward and rest your head on the block. By placing the head on a block, we de-stimulate the brain and activate the third eye. This leads to a more relaxed, meditative, and peaceful sensation.

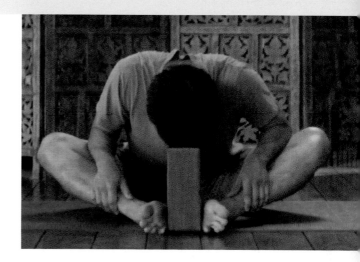

## 3. Sphinx Pose (*Salamba Bhujangasana*)

Lie on your belly and prop yourself up on your forearms. Place your elbows directly under your shoulders and spread your fingers wide, hands aligned with elbows and pressed into the floor. Your legs extend straight back behind you with your toenails on the floor. Press the legs down as if imprinting them in sand, and slightly engage your lower belly. Pressing into the arms, slide your chest slightly forward and up. Your focus point (*drishti*) is directly in front of you, with your chin level with the ground (**a**). This pose is very calming and gently uplifting.

Hold for 5–10 breaths, then rest in Crocodile Pose by releasing down onto your belly, turning your toes out, and letting your heels fall in (**b**). If this feels very unnatural to you and uncomfortable, switch it around (toes in, heels out). Cross your arms so that your fingertips come near your elbows, and place your forehead on your forearms.

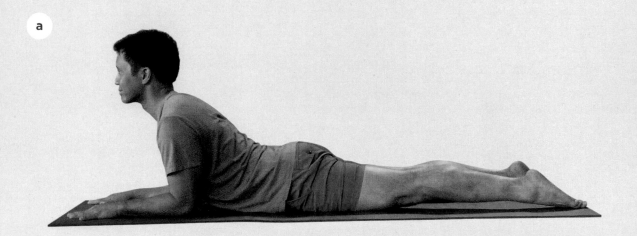

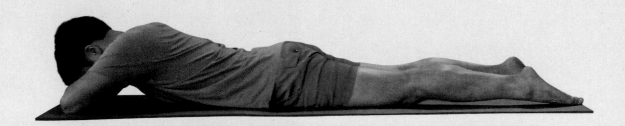

# Trust

## OR BUST

One mantra has stayed with me for as long as I can remember—trust. It may be to trust myself and my intuition (which is a lifelong practice); it may be to trust that the universe is benign and all is unfolding as it should; and it may be to trust the larger picture even if I can't see it right now. Trust is a true combination of action and surrender. We must *will* ourselves to *allow* ourselves to relax into trust. When my trust gets shaky or falters, I consider its opposite— a life of suspicion, doubt, and unease. To activate the aspects of willpower and surrender we will work with three energy centers: the heart, the solar plexus, and the third eye.

### 1. Mudra for Unshakable Trust (*Vajrapradama*)

This sequence works with the breath and the mudra to create a rhythm that balances and engages the solar plexus and heart chakras. *Vajra* means "thunderbolt," which in yoga represents powerful and focused energy and in Buddhism is seen as a weapon against self-doubt.

Sit cross-legged in *Sukhasana* or *Siddhasana* (page 10) or on the edge of a chair. Interlace your fingers, facing your chest, and a few inches away from heart center (**a**). Keep the elbows slightly lifted and release physical and mental tension by following your breath for

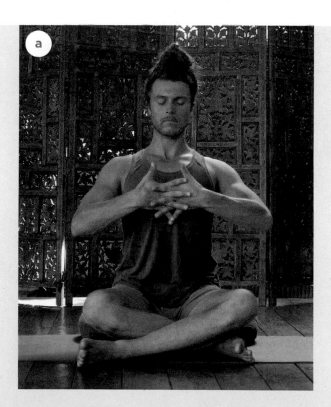

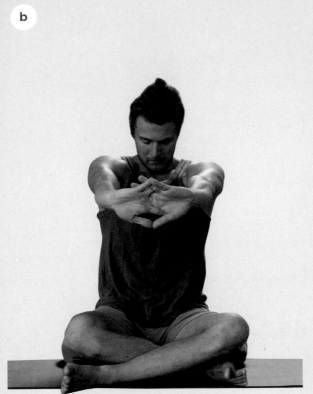

b

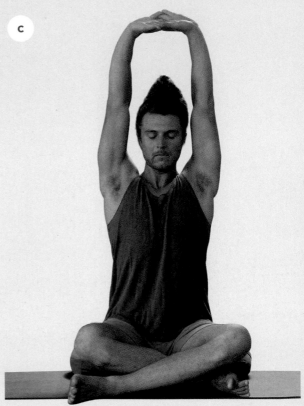

c

a few moments. Inhale deeply, and as you exhale flip your hands and push them forward, rounding your upper back and engaging your belly button. Release your head toward your heart (**b**).

Inhale and lift your arms up, still with your hands interlaced and now facing the sky (**c**). Inhale there, and as you exhale come back to the rounding of the upper back and drawing the belly in with your palms facing out in front of you. With your next inhale flip the hands, coming back to a straight spine and your arms and hands in the starting position. Hold there

for as many breaths as you like and then begin the sequence with the breath again. Repeat 3–5 times, resting in between.

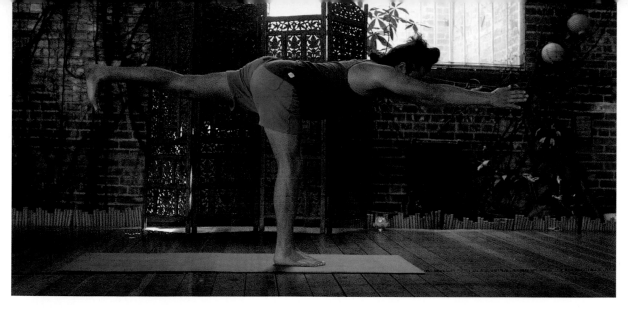

## 2. Warrior III (*Virabhadrasana III*)

Change is often a precursor to lack of trust. Grounding yourself while simultaneously practicing surrender can be a powerful antidote. Balancing asanas are a perfect recipe.

Start in *Tadasana* (page 9) and step or hop your feet wide apart (approximately 4 feet/ 1.25 meters). Follow the instructions on pages 96–97 to come into Warrior I. Stay in Warrior I for a few breaths.

Then pivot to the ball of your left foot and shift your weight over your right leg. Step your back foot up toward your bent leg as needed and move your weight completely to the right leg, lifting the left behind you to hip height. Stretch your arms in front of you dynamically. Keep your abdominal muscles firm and flex your left foot so that the toes point to the floor. Your focus point (*drishti*) can be a few feet beyond your toes, at eye height or on the ground. Try to keep your hips square, and don't lock your right knee.

Stay for 3–5 breaths, then step back to Warrior I. Rest in *Tadasana* before switching to the other side. Trust that you can balance with your strength and your ease, and should you fall, let go with grace and humor.

**Modifications:** For tender backs or to build your strength for this pose, come into it as described above and instead of stretching your arms in front, place your hands on two blocks on the floor, directly under your shoulders (**below**). Another option is to come into Warrior I roughly 4 feet (1.25 meters) from a wall and then, as you shift into Warrior III, place your hands on the wall for support at shoulder height. The elbows may be bent.

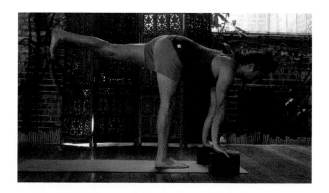

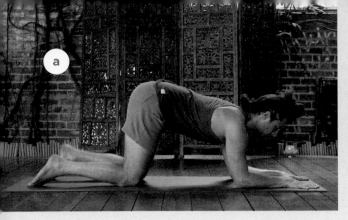

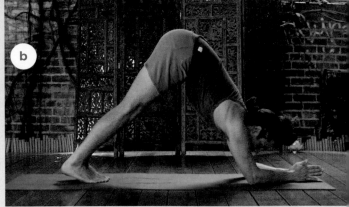

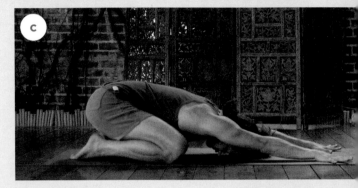

### 3. Dolphin Pose (*Ardha Pincha Mayurasana*) with Child's Pose (*Adho Mukha Virasana*)

The third eye (the sixth chakra, *Ajna*) can be activated with poses that encourage prana to flow in that direction, or have the third eye placed upon something, or through meditation. We will start with an inversion, Dolphin Pose. In addition to awakening the third eye, Dolphin Pose opens the shoulders, tones the abdomen, and strengthens the entire body.

Begin on hands and knees. Place your forearms on the floor with your shoulders directly over your elbows (**a**), and keep your hands in line with your elbows. Tuck your toes under, pull in your belly button, and lift up your hips as you press into the floor with your arms. Keep the knees bent to start and then as you exhale, slowly straighten your legs and press your chest toward your thighs, as you do in Downward Dog. You will be in the shape of the letter A (**b**, showing variation). Try to keep your upper back flat, and if that is not possible, bend your knees a little. Upper body flexibility will come in time. You can let your head hang, or lift it slightly and gaze a few inches in front of you in the direction of your fingertips. Send

your attention to the space between your eyebrows (*Ajna*), and visualize your breath coming into the third eye as the color indigo. Hold for 3–5 breaths, then come into Child's Pose with your big toes together and your knees apart (**c**). Rest your forehead on the floor and continue with the meditation of the indigo breath.

**Variation:** Follow the same directions, but with your hands pressed together in a prayer position so that the edges of your hands are pressing into the floor. Lift your head so that your gaze is toward the space where the base of your palms meet (**b**). Breathe the indigo breath here.

**Modification:** If you like, you can go straight into Child's Pose, directing your attention to the *Ajna* chakra and the indigo-colored breath.

# Acceptance

## THE GATEWAY TO CHANGE

Ironically, when we seek change, that's often the time when it may appear to be elusive, and this is where acceptance can be a deceptively active choice. If we can become more comfortable with the natural and dynamic law that life is always changing and so are we, we can lean into the flow of change and become inspired by possibility and the opportunity to grow—and to grow is our ultimate true nature. By accepting what is in this moment, without knee-jerk reactions, we free ourselves to move like water, fluid, flexible, always changing as the terrain does. We accept what comes our way, adapt, and transform. Think of how water changes the stones that it flows over. Life changes us, and if we can accept rather than resist the moment we are in, we may find the changes we are actually looking for.

### 1. Pick Your Pose!

Here you are going to choose a pose that is particularly challenging for you because of those pesky hips, crunchy shoulders, or stubborn hamstrings! And then there's always the balancing poses, which can test even the most accepting person on occasion. If you are the "can't sit still" type, go straight for seated meditation. So choose your nemesis pose and take the precaution of doing a proper warm-up if necessary (pages 16–22).

Once in your pose, hold it and breathe and practice not resisting. That means physically not struggling or fidgeting and mentally not engaging in distracting commentary and opinions. Instead, focus on breathing and being present. If your mind is like a tiger in a cage, say to yourself, "This is what's happening," and then come back to the sound and feeling of your breath. Practice acceptance and observe if you feel your body and mind shift, release, transform. Even a little bit of acceptance can go a long way.

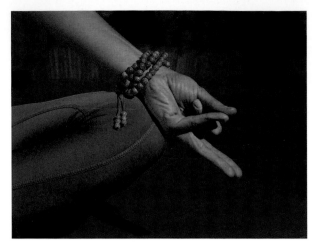

## 2. Acceptance Mudra

Sit cross-legged in *Sukhasana* or *Siddhasana* (page 10) or on a chair. Bring the index finger of each hand to the base of your thumb. Place the thumb of each hand to the inner, lower corner of your pinky fingernail or to the pad of the pinky finger. Your middle and ring fingers extend away from your palm. Close your eyes. As in your nemesis pose, keep your awareness with your breath and the experience of being rather than doing. Let your breath wash over you as water does over stones, and allow yourself to feel the peace and strength of accepting yourself, your life, your circumstances. Remember that everything changes and if you don't obstruct the flow, you can become the butterfly, even in the middle of a storm.

## 3. Dirga Breath in *Savasana*

Lie on your back, arms out from your sides, palms up, fingers curling naturally, in *Savasana* (page 13). Relax and close your eyes. Inhale into the bottom of your belly, then your solar plexus, and finish the breath in your chest. You may find it helpful to visualize filling a glass with water from bottom to top. Pause briefly when you have filled your glass and then exhale from the upper chest, solar plexus, and finally the bottom of the belly, as if you were pouring the water from the glass. Continue with *Dirga* (also known as Three Part) Breath for 1–3 minutes.

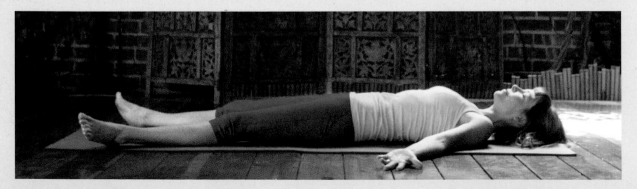

# Creativity

## YOU ARE THE ARTIST AND THE ART

You don't need to be a professional, or even fledgling, artist to desire some spark in the arena of creativity. We all long to feel the flow of creation move through us as parents, mates, workers, adventurers, seekers, and writers of our own story. The second chakra (*Svadhisthana*) is the energetic center for both creativity and pleasure, and it's no coincidence that these emanate from the same place. It is pleasurable to create. This is the sacral chakra, and it involves stuck energy in the hips. So let's loosen up and let that river of creativity flow!

### 1. Swirling Butterfly Pose (*Baddha Konasana*)

Sit on the floor, spine straight, knees out to the sides, and the soles of your feet together. Hold your ankles and move your body in circles, beginning clockwise. As you move toward your feet, inhale and let your belly expand. As you move your torso away from your feet, exhale and contract your belly. Swirl for 8 circles in each direction. When finished, hold Butterfly Pose for 5 more breaths, relaxing your belly.

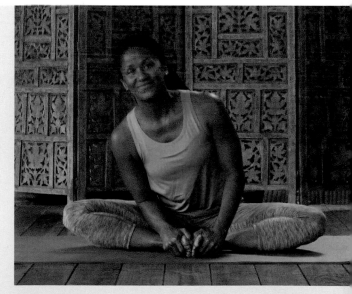

**Modification:** The expansion and contraction of the belly with the breath is a variation on nauli (turning the abdominal muscles), which is a cleansing yogic exercise (*kriya*). While it can be very useful for digestion and unblocking energy in the second and third chakras (sacral and solar plexus), if it becomes too tiring or you have trouble with it, just relax into your breath as you move.

## 2. Frog Pose (*Mandukasana*)

For this pose you will need some padding under your knees—a yoga mat plus blankets if necessary.

Come to tabletop position, hands under your shoulders and knees at hip-width. Then come down onto your forearms with your palms flat on the floor. Separate your knees so they are as wide apart as is comfortable, flex your feet and place their inner edges on the floor. Your ankles should be in direct line with your knees, with the feet turned out to the side. If you wish, you can place your hands in prayer position.

Breathe here for a few moments, and if you can't feel much of a stretch in your inner thighs, groin, and hips, begin to ease your hips back toward your feet, maintaining the alignment of your knees and ankles. Some people may have a more satisfying experience taking the hips slightly forward. Keep your abdomen engaged so your lower back is protected. Your face is toward the floor, or gaze directed slightly ahead, and your shoulders are away from your ears.

Take 5–8 breaths, visualizing as blocks of ice melting any place in the lower body where you feel stuck or tight. Remember that when the ice melts, spring comes and a potpourri of colorful creativity emerges.

To come out of the pose, come onto your hands and slowly bring the legs toward each other with strong inner thighs and a firm abdomen. Once the legs are together, spend a few moments in Child's Pose with the legs together (*Balasana*, page 12).

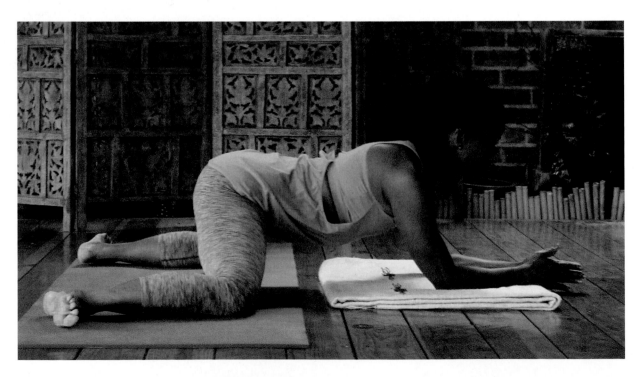

### 3. Break of Day Mudra (*Ushas Mudra*) with Skull Shining (*Kapalabhati*) Breath

*Ushas Mudra* is one of my favorites. As well as Break of Day, it is known as the Origin of Good Things Mudra. It lifts the energy and unleashes creative impulses. It brings the energy from the lower chakras up to the higher chakras and can enhance our ability to experience pleasure.

Sit cross-legged in *Sukhasana* or *Siddhasana* (page 10) or on a chair. Interlace your fingers with the palms facing slightly upward. For women, encircle the right thumb with the left thumb and index finger. For men, encircle the left thumb with the right thumb and index finger. Relax your shoulders, bend your elbows, and hold the mudra just below your navel and a few inches from your body.

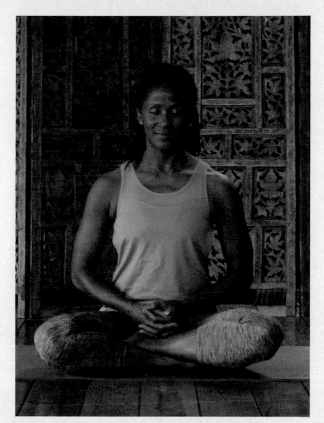

Begin your Skull Shining Breath, by inhaling fully through your nose and exhaling through your mouth. On your next inhale, stop short of a full breath and exhale through your nose with a forceful blow as your abdomen engages toward your navel. Let your inhale naturally follow. The focus is on the exhale, which comes from the action of the belly pulling in. The inhale is a slow, natural reaction to the force of the exhale. Both breaths are done through the nose.

Practice 1–3 rounds of Skull Shining Breath. When you are finished, sit quietly with the mudra and enjoy the spark of inspiration that is the light of your creativity shining from within.

# Appreciation and Gratitude

## THIS IS WHERE HAPPY LIVES

Gratitude is taking the time to honor who and what we hold dear and to count our blessings. As a practice, it is life-changing. Appreciation has its own nuance. There is almost nothing as life-shifting as stopping in your tracks to appreciate. It can take a dark mood and bring in the light in a heartbeat. To recognize that we live in this remarkable atmosphere is an awe-inspiring gift. Sometimes these feelings come effortlessly, but there are moments when we must remember and practice being receptive. When we do endeavor consciously to live in a space of appreciation and gratitude, it can soften bad news, hard moments, and scary times and open our hearts and minds to the bounty of love and exquisiteness that surrounds us. Before practicing the following sequence, I suggest that you do 5–10 rounds of Sun Salutations (pages 16–22).

## 1. Reverse Warrior (*Viparita Virabhadrasana*)

From *Tadasana* (page 9), follow the instructions on page 98 to come into Warrior II (**a**), leading with your left leg. Hold for 3 breaths.

Turn your palms up, and notice your heart lift and open. Inhale and lengthen upward through the crown of your head, making your spine long. Then reach back with your right hand and place the palm on your right thigh. Stretch your left arm up to the sky and then arch back, with your left bicep a few inches from your left ear. You can stay facing to the side, or, if your back allows, you can twist your face and chest upward (**b**). Avoid putting pressure on the right leg, but rather keep a light touch with the palm and let the legs do the work. Like a tree, grow roots through your feet and let your heart open like a flower. Hold for 3–5 breaths and repeat on the other side.

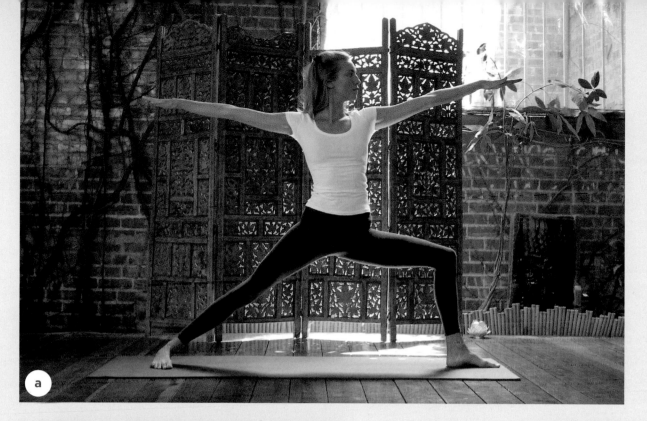

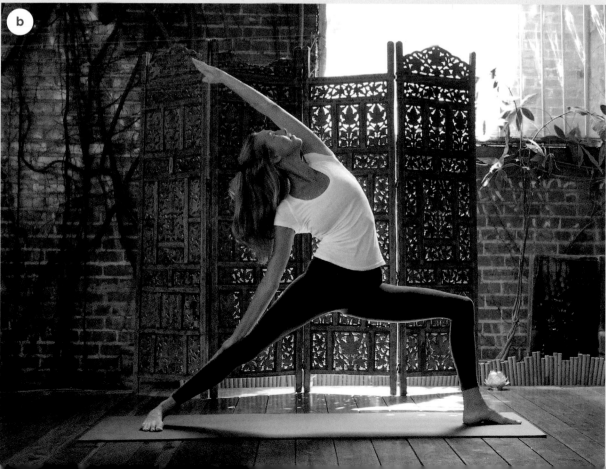

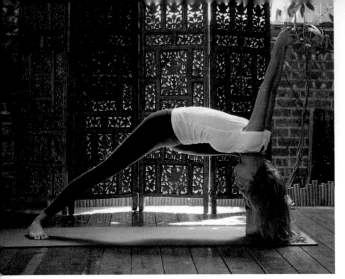

facing in, and roll your shoulders in toward each other. Move your right foot a couple of inches to the right. Stay grounded through the left heel as you lift your face and chest to the sky, inhale, and then bow down inside the left leg. Your head is hovering above the floor and your arms are reaching away from your back toward the sky. Hug the thighs toward each other and engage your abdominal muscles. Breathe and relax into this humble, dynamic asana for 3–5 breaths, then switch sides.

**Variation:** If you like, you can go from Reverse Warrior (previous page) to Humble Warrior before changing sides.

**Modification:** Instead of interlacing the fingers behind you, place your forearms on a chair or blocks and bring the hands together in prayer position.

### 2. Humble Warrior (*Baddha Virabhadrasana*)

From *Tadasana* (page 9), follow the instructions on pages 96–97 to come into Warrior I, leading with your left leg. Hold for 3 breaths.

Then, maintaining the lower half of the pose, interlace your fingers behind your back, palms

### 3. Cross-legged Pose (*Sukhasana*) or Thunderbolt Pose (*Vajrasana*) with *Atmanjali Mudra*

Sit either cross-legged in *Sukhasana* (page 10) or on your shins with your sitting bones on the soles of your feet (Thunderbolt Pose), and bring your hands together in front of your heart center, but not touching the body as in *Anjali Mudra*. The fingers and base of the palms touch each other but keep an open space in the center of the palms. Lean a few inches forward with the head bowed. This position allows the heart energy to pour right into the hands, and softens the ego to submerge into a state of deep, peaceful gratitude. Stay as long as you like with easy breaths.

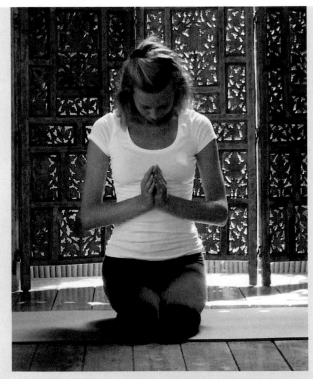

# Abundance

## ANOTHER HELPING, PLEASE

When we think of abundance in only practical, material terms, we tend to focus on the *having* rather than the *being*, which turns our attention to lack and fear of loss. When we touch upon the infinite nature of abundance, we feel the potential in each moment to experience appreciation for what is and to awaken to the understanding that there is never a scarcity of anything. There is only a block to the channel by which we create and allow its manifestation to become known to us. Fear and clinging cut off our ability to flow, create, and receive. Let's tap into acknowledging all that is abundant here and now, and when that energy has been activated, make our request for further illumination along the path of abundance. Before beginning this sequence, I suggest practicing 5-10 rounds of Sun Salutations (pages 16–22). Choose whichever one you feel like.

### 1. Upward Plank Pose (*Purvottanasana*)

To start, sit on the floor in *Dandasana* (page 9)—legs outstretched, feet flexed, spine straight, shoulders back and down, hands by your hips, fingers facing forward. Place your hands 6-8 inches (15-20 centimeters) behind you, fingers still facing forward, and lean back. Point your toes, engage your legs, and push into the floor with your hands as you lift your hips and torso. Squeeze the legs together and reach for the floor with your toes.

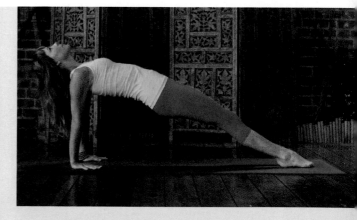

Slowly, keeping your neck long, extend your head back.

Breathe here, imagining all the bounty and abundance in your life sitting right on your abdomen like a table set for a feast. Keep your chest high, heart open, and breath steady for 3–5 breaths. Come down and rest, hugging your knees into your chest (page 13).

**Modification:** If this is too strenuous or you have a problem with wrists, shoulders, or back, go for an upward tabletop position instead. Get as far as leaning back and then place your feet under your bent knees and lift up.

## 2. Wild Thing (*Camatkarasana*)

When we begin to access a feeling of the infinite potential in each moment, many a surprise or miracle can occur, and Wild Thing is also known as Surprise or Miracle Pose.

From Downward Dog (page 11), follow the instructions on pages 101–102 to come into Plank (**a**).

Shift your weight to the right hand and roll onto the outer edge of the right foot as you would for Side Plank (page 103) (**b**).

Step your left foot back with the knee bent, and place the foot on the floor. Extend your left arm over your head, reaching back, and extend the right leg, pointing the toe (**c**).

Take 3–5 breaths here and allow yourself to experience a feeling of openness and faith.

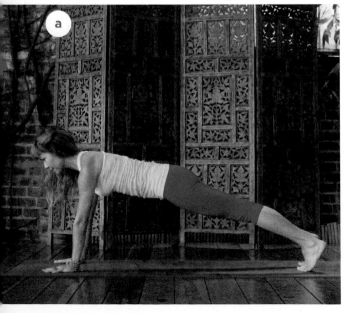

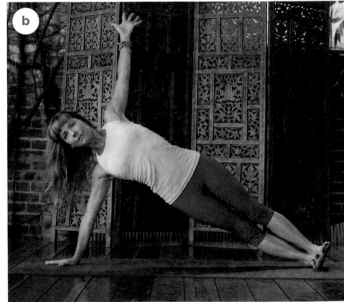

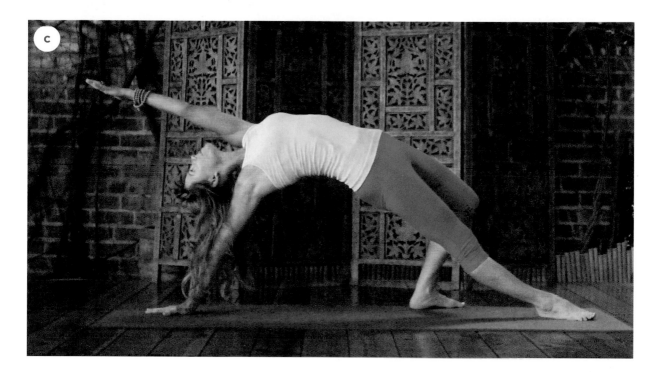

### 3. *Lakshmi* Full Moon Mudra

This is especially powerful at the full moon, but can be done any time! Sit on the floor with the soles of your feet together. If this is too much without support, lean against a wall. Bring your hands side by side with the pinkies touching and extended. Curl in the index, middle, and ring fingers, but not so much as to touch the palm. Relax and release tension in the body and soften into this cradle of receiving. Welcome the creativity and light of your spirit to reflect back to you the abundance that is so keenly present in your life already. Offer your heart and service to the preservation and expansion of this infinite universe, and ask for what you need to stay tuned in to a grateful attitude and to manifest your deepest desires

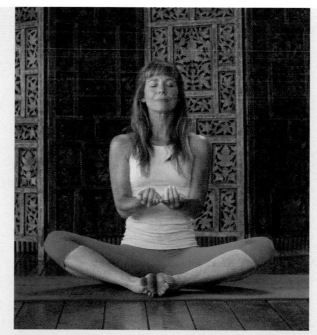

for the good of all concerned. Stay here, breathing peacefully, knowingly, trustingly, for as long as you like.

# Balance

## EMBRACE THE JUGGLING ACT

Balance, like juggling, is a dynamic act. The urge is to overorganize our lives into a rigid idea of balance, but this can then overwhelm us. However, we can reach for a deeper center and follow our instincts. Even with endless demands and responsibilities, we can artfully practice catching the balls with a smile. When we do fall, or drop the ball, we can display a sense of humor and move on. Practice staying spontaneous, flexible, and connected to NOW and watch your schedule and your energy align.

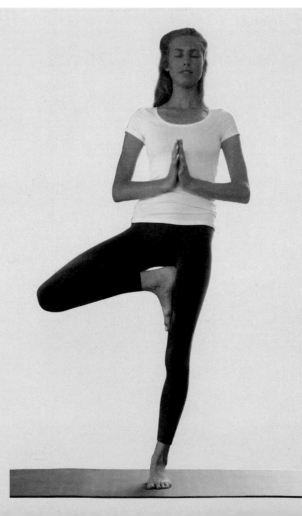

### 1. Tree Pose (*Vrksasana*) with Closed Eyes

Follow the instructions on pages 84–85 to get into Tree Pose. When stable, place your hands in prayer position at heart center (*Anjali Mudra*).

Now close your eyes and move your gaze within. We tend to rely on our vision for much of our balance in the world, both physically and emotionally, by responding to external stimuli and reacting to what we see. When we let go of finding our footing based on what is surrounding us, we naturally drop into an inner center. While it may feel much less stable or sure-footed, the practice here is to relax into the wobble and sway, rather than to cling to the pose or rigid mind-set. Finding balance can often come from being willing to let go and even fall. Find your edge in the pose, that turning point where holding on and letting go meet, like the sun passing the moon on its way to dawn.

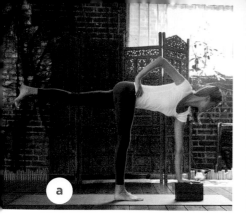
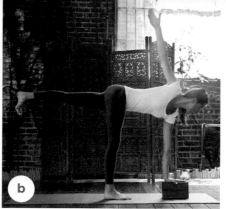
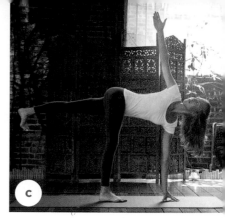

## 2. Revolved Half Moon (*Parivrtta Ardha Chandrasana*)

Begin by standing tall in *Tadasana* (page 9). Place your hands on your hips and jump or step your feet wide apart (approximately 4 feet/ 1.25 meters). Turn your left foot in by about 60 degrees and your right foot out by 90 degrees, and face forward over your right leg. Extend your arms out to the sides at shoulder height.

Inhale, and as you exhale, twist so that your left arm is reaching forward and your right arm is reaching back. Inhale, and as you exhale, bring your left hand to the floor or onto a block underneath your left shoulder and your right hand to your hip. Shift your weight completely to your right leg and lift your left leg off the floor (**a**). Stretch your right arm up directly over your shoulder and gaze either down toward the floor (**b**) or up toward your right thumb (**c**). Reach in every direction, and keep the back leg lifted to hip height and actively stretching.

Attempt to expand and radiate energy even as you find the soft side of the asana—the magical place where sun and moon meet.

## 3. Alternate Nostril Breathing (*Nadi Shodhana*)

This pranayama technique clears the two main energy channels of the body and balances the hemispheres of the brain, which can result in greater energy and focus. Follow the instructions on page 89.

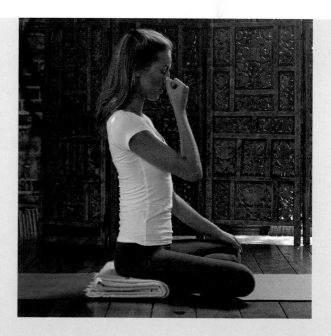

# Energy

## HARNESS YOUR MOST PRECIOUS RESOURCE

Energy—more precious than gold, at times more elusive than world peace, something we are born with in abundance and tend to appreciate and long for much more as we grow older. Fortunately, yoga can not only increase our energy but also balance it, so that we avoid those mysterious peaks and valleys and ease into a sustained groove of flowing life force. In this definition, the intention is not continuously to grasp for some peak experience of boundless physical stamina, but to feel the spark of prana guiding us from a deeper source. It is closer to inspiration than animation. When we practice yoga, we open our energy channels (*nadis*, of which there are many thousands), and this brings a state of awakening that sparks the life-affirming energy of the sun and the luminescence and ease of the moon. A Sanskrit word for this is *sattvic*. It is the balance of energy that brings lightness.

### 1. Skull Shining Breath (*Kapalabhati*)

This pranayama is well named, because it is quite possible that you will glow when you are finished. It purifies the frontal brain, tones the abdominals, aids in digestion, oxygenates the blood, and clears the mind.

Sit on the floor in *Sukhasana* or *Siddhasana* (page 10), or on a chair with your feet flat on the ground. Take *Jnana Mudra* with the thumb and index fingers touching to form a circle and the arms extended. Inhale fully through

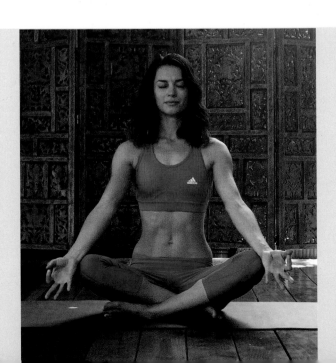

your nose and exhale through your mouth. On your next inhale, stop short of a full breath and exhale through your nose with a forceful blow as your abdomen engages toward your navel. Let your inhale follow naturally. The focus in this practice is on the exhale, which comes from the action of the belly pulling in. The inhale is a slow, natural reaction to the force of the exhale. Both breaths are done through the nose.

For beginners, practice 3 rounds of 11 with 2–3 natural breaths in between. If you are a seasoned practitioner, you can increase to 3 rounds of 27. When you are finished, sit quietly, breathing slowly for a few minutes, and bask in your raised vibration.

## 2. Sun Salutation Variation (*Surya Namaskar B*)

This mini vinyasa flow sequence is described in full on pages 16–17, and is sure to get your juices flowing.

## 3. Bridge Pose (*Setu Bandhasana*) or Bow Pose (*Dhanurasana*)

Follow the instructions on page 60 to come into Bridge Pose (**right**). Breathe 5 deep, slow breaths before slowly rolling down from the top vertebrae to the bottom. Rest in Reclining Butterfly in between poses by lying on your back with the soles of the feet together, one hand on your heart and one hand on your belly. When you are finished, hug the knees to the chest and make slow circles to massage the low back.

For Bow Pose (**below right**), follow the instructions on page 114.

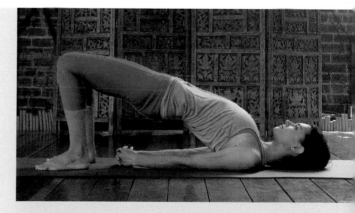

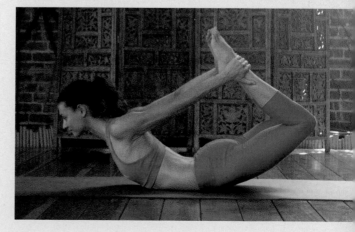

# Confidence

## FEEL YOUR POWER

To be in tune with the deepest layer of confidence and power is to cultivate and nurture a belief in oneself—a belief that has taken root based on experience, mistakes that you have allowed yourself to make, and the knowledge that your authenticity is what the world needs and desires of you. When we seek true confidence and allow ourselves to develop into our unique and essential self, we align ourselves with the energy of source. The solar plexus is the physical center for confidence and joy. We will activate and balance the second chakra (*Manipura*) to connect to that place within where we remember our worth and enjoy playing with powerful creativity as we shape our world. Before beginning the following sequence, practice 5–10 rounds of Sun Salutations (pages 16–22).

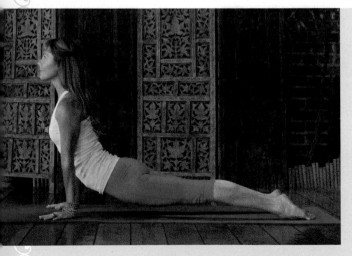

### 1. Upward Facing Dog (*Urdhva Mukha Svanasana*)

This pose strengthens the entire body, opens the heart, stretches the core, and inspires a feeling of confidence. It's important to be properly aligned to avoid discomfort or even injury.

Lie prone with the tops of your feet on the floor and place your hands, palms down, alongside your waist. Your elbows are bent and your triceps parallel with the floor. As you inhale, push down into the ground and pull your chest forward, straightening your arms. Only your hands and the tops of your feet remain on the floor. Push strongly into the ground with your feet so that your legs are charged, and keep your belly firm. Lift up through the chest and draw your shoulder blades into your back. Your focus point (*drishti*) can be straight ahead or up toward the sky, as long as you keep your neck long when taking the head back. If your wrists are a bit weak, press just the very tips of your fingerpads into the floor to engage the arms and take pressure off the wrist joints. Hold for 3–4 breaths and then ease your way down and rest. Repeat 1–3 times.

**Modification:** If you have a back, wrist, or shoulder injury that is relatively fresh, it would be wise to opt for Cobra Pose (pages 43–44) instead.

## 2. Crow Pose (*Bakasana*)

While Crow Pose—also known as Crane Pose—can be a big challenge to the ego, it can also be the most satisfying of accomplishments because you end up taking flight, and defying gravity is always fun. As with all poses, but especially this one, try to take it one breath at a time and not become too distracted by the final goal. Everything happens in its own time, as I am sure every baby bird can attest. If you are a more seasoned bird, feel free to enjoy any variations on this arm balance that tickle your fancy.

There are several ways to approach the pose. Let's begin from the ground up. Come into Garland Pose (page 48)—squat with your feet close together and your knees wider than your hips. Rest your heels on a rolled-up blanket or block if they don't touch the floor. Move your torso between your knees and take hold of your ankles, using your elbows to keep your hips open.

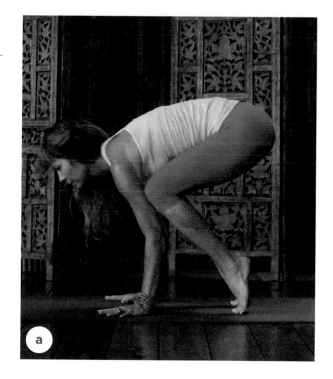

Now place your hands in front of you on the ground. Lift your rear and bend your elbows back toward you. Shift your weight forward, placing your knees on your upper arms as close to the armpits as possible. Keep your head lifted and gaze a couple feet in front of you. Come onto your tippy toes (**a**),

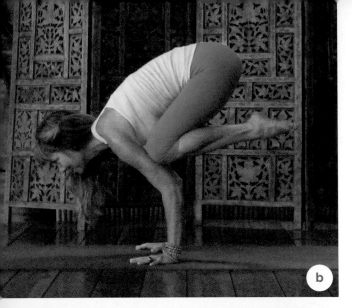

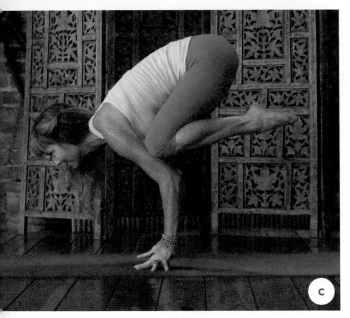

Now lift one or both feet off the ground as you squeeze your pelvic floor and perineum (*Mula Bandha* Lock) (**b**). Engage your abdominals, pulling them up and in to dome your back (*Uddiyana Bandha* Lock). Make sure you keep your hands either flat on the floor or in a cat claw with the tips of your fingerpads pressing down (**c**). Elbows should be drawing in, arms straightening, and the hands pressing down. As the belly lifts up, you will feel less pressure on your arms. It may take some practice to defy gravity, but it can happen, and the pose can eventually feel light rather than heavy. Relax, breathe, and enjoy the process whether you take flight or set the foundation for future flights!

**Modifications:** If you are having trouble getting liftoff, you can place a block or books beneath your feet so that you start from a perch. If you are especially afraid of your face hitting the floor (understandable!), place a block beneath your head (**below left**) and, once your feet are off the floor, lift your head. You may also have greater success by bringing your legs lower down and outside of your arms, and squeezing your legs strongly into your arms.

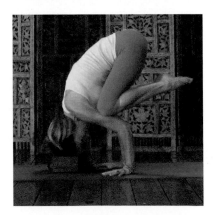

### 3. Empty Lake Bed Mudra (*Tadaka Mudra*)

This whole-body mudra is a wonderful way to get the digestive fires burning. It tones the abdomen and helps to release tension there, and can be detoxifying for the organs.

Lie on your back, interlace your fingers, and as you inhale, stretch the arms overhead with your palms facing away from your head. Let your abdomen expand with the breath. When you exhale, release your chin toward your chest (head still on the floor), and draw your ribs and navel in toward the floor as your chest lifts higher toward your chin. Pause for a few moments after the exhale and then repeat for 4–6 breaths.

**Variation:** Add *Matangi Mudra* to enhance the effects of toning, harmonizing, and improved digestion. This mudra can also increase confidence and boost self-esteem. Interlace the fingers except for the middle fingers, which extend, and proceed as before. Alternatively, take a comfortable seated position and hold the mudra at your navel with the fingers pointing toward your chin.

**Modification:** If you want a less-is-more moment here, this restorative backbend may hit the spot and relax your third chakra (*Manipura*), the solar plexus. Place a bolster or stack of folded blankets lengthwise and sit in the middle of it. Lie back so that the bottom edge of your shoulder blades (roughly the bra-strap line) is on the support and your head and shoulders are on the floor. You can add a blanket for your head or rolled under your neck if you like. Your legs will extend off your support. If this feels too much for your lower back, roll a towel or blanket under your ankles or place two blocks there and allow your feet to float free. Place your hands in *Matangi Mudra* for 1 minute before relaxing your arms to your sides.

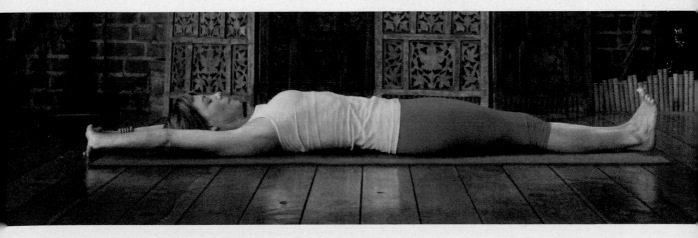

# Grounding

## FIND YOUR ROOTS

We are at our best when our life force has clear channels through which to flow and a path to follow. The origins of the path are the foundations, the secure roots from which we begin, expand, and ultimately flower. Think of any plant—the roots must be nourished with water and food before it can break through and receive the sun and air to complete its lifecycle. We can ground ourselves by focusing on our essential beliefs, caring for our home, and tending to our basic survival needs with love and attention rather than resentment and fear. As you move through this sequence, consider what seeds are taking root in your foundation and what has already provided you with inspiration and security.

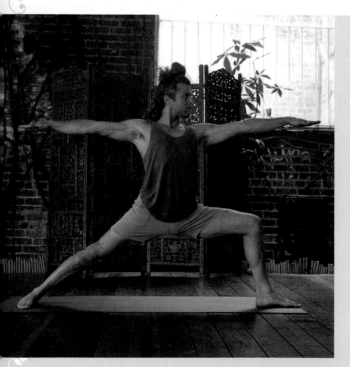

### 1. Warrior II (*Virabhadrasana II*)

Follow the instructions on page 98 to come into Warrior II. Engage your abdominals and hold for 3–5 breaths. On an inhale, lift out of the pose and rest your hands on your hips. Turn your feet to the other side and repeat.

## 2. Horse Stance with *Ujjayi* Breath

There is no agreed Sanskrit term for this asana, but there is nothing shaky about it other than possibly your thighs! Start in *Tadasana* (page 9), place your hands on your hips, and step your feet wide apart (approximately 4 feet/ 1.25 meters). Turn your toes out and bend your knees until your thighs are parallel, or close to parallel, to the ground. Lengthen your tailbone toward the floor and draw your belly button in. Extend your arms straight overhead with the palms facing each other.

Hold the pose for 30 seconds to 1 minute while taking *Ujjayi* breaths (page 28). Inhale through your nose while lightly constricting your throat so that your breath makes a "whoosh" sound. Exhale in the same manner, listening for that sound.

Repeat the pose 3 times, resting in *Tadasana* or Standing Forward Fold (page 11) in between.

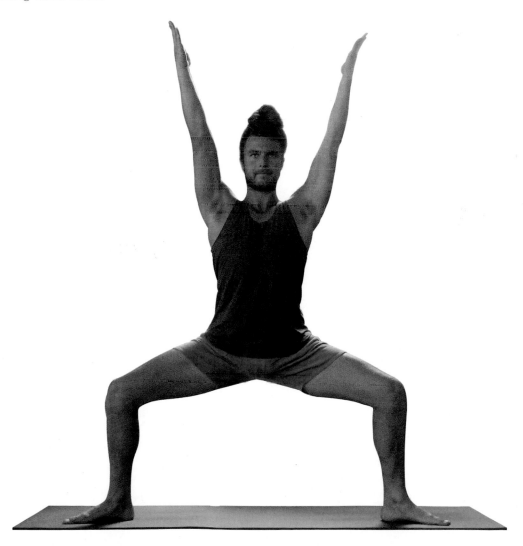

**Variations:** After practicing one round as described above, you may wish to play with these variations.

Place both hands on your thighs with your fingers pointing down. Inhale, and then as you exhale, twist to one side, looking over the same shoulder and keeping the thighs open. Repeat on the other side.

Place one forearm on your thigh and stretch the opposite arm overhead, lengthening the torso and side waist. Hold for 30 seconds and repeat on the other side.

This one requires a lot of hip flexibility, so be mindful and ease into it to see how your body responds. Place one hand on the floor and stretch the other arm straight up to the sky, turning your face and torso toward your extended arm. Hold for 30 seconds and repeat on the other side.

## 3. *Prithvi Mudra*

Sit on the ground in a comfortable meditation position. Bring your thumb and ring finger together on each hand. Sit tall and stretch your arms out by your sides with the fingers touching the floor. Imagine your spine lifting skyward on the inhale and your energy lifting with it (**a**). On your exhale, stay lifted and imagine roots growing from every part of your body that is touching the floor. Feel the gentle tug as you connect more deeply to earth energy. Let it nourish and center you for 5 breaths. Then, maintaining the mudra, turn the hands to face up and place them with the arms extended on your legs (**b**). Hold for another 1–3 minutes.

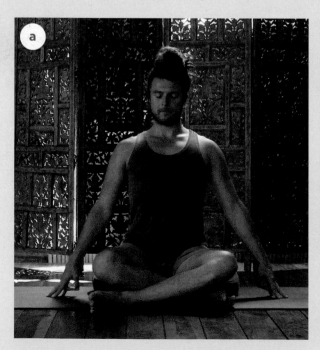

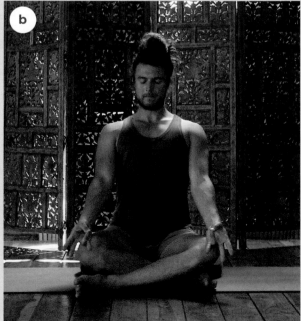

# Connection

## YOU ARE DIVINE

No matter what our spiritual beliefs may be, it is not too difficult to imagine that we share a common home, this planet Earth, and that we spring from a common source. To have a connection to something beyond ourselves is to experience belonging and support, and to diminish feelings of isolation. When we see an unconditional source of vitality and love running through all living things, we recognize that it runs through us. We see more clearly that we are essential, universal, and unique. Not only is this world a place for us to explore, but also its magnificence is part of us. If we can stay in touch with our own divine essence, we have endless source energy at our fingertips with which we can shape the world into its most harmonious, peaceful, and vibrant manifestation.

### 1. Rabbit Pose (*Sasangasana*)

The top of the head is the physical center for the seventh chakra, the crown (*Sahasrara*). This pose activates the chakra and relieves mental tension.

Begin in Child's Pose (*Balasana*)—from hands and knees, draw your navel in and sit back on your heels with knees together. Take your arms back toward your feet. Set your forehead on the floor, with your chin tucked in. Reach back and wrap your hands around the outside of your feet (**a**).

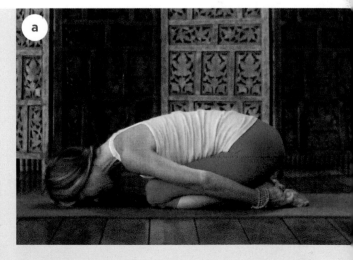

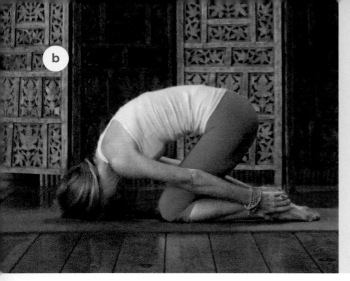

As you inhale, roll toward the crown of your head with your back rounded and your legs strong (**b**). Hold for 3–5 breaths and then roll back down and rest in Child's Pose. Repeat 1–3 times.

## 2. *Uttarabodhi Mudra*

Sit cross-legged on the floor in *Sukhasana* or *Siddhasana* (page 10), or on a chair, and interlace all your fingers except for the index fingers, which point upward. Cross your thumbs and lift your arms over your head so that your hands are a few inches from the crown, elbows bent. As if you are a human divining rod, breathe in the electric energy of the universe and draw its light into your body, mind, and spirit. Hold for 1–3 minutes (**a**). If your arms become tired or you feel pain or extreme tension, maintain the mudra and bring it to the peak of your ribcage in front of you (**b**).

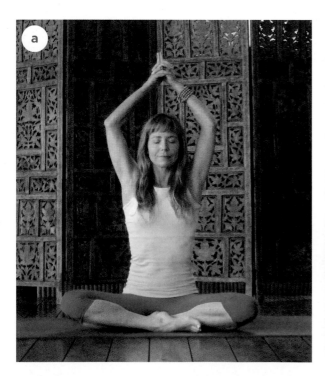

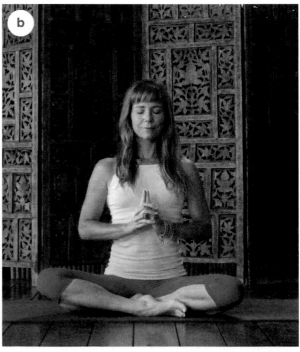

### 3. Chant *Om*

Sit comfortably with your hands relaxed naturally or in *Jnana Mudra* with the thumb and index finger touching. Close your eyes. Bring your third eye—the sixth chakra, the space between your eyebrows (*Ajna*)—into your awareness. Take a few moments focusing on that point. You may even be able to visualize the color indigo or a shade of purple there. When you feel ready, begin to chant "Ohhhmmm ..."

The mantra of *Om* is said to represent everything from the most infinitesimal aspect of creation to the most omnipotent. As with all yoga practice, this is not a religious mantra.

It is an invocation, an honoring of the seed of creation, and represents our life journey, all that came before, and all that comes after. Its full symbolism is displayed when written as

**A** *Ahhh*: the beginning, or energy of creation.

**U** *Ooohh*: maintaining, or energy of sustaining.

**M** *Mmmm*: the deconstruction, or energy of transformation.

When we chant and contemplate "*om*," we are opening to a deeper sense of being. After all, we are human *beings*; we are not human *doings*.

Namaste!

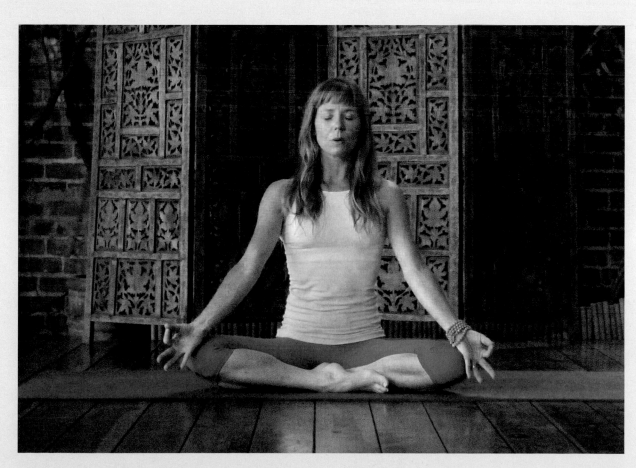

# PART 4

# Complete Mini Sequences

## FOR EVERYDAY PRACTICE

This section offers three sequences for morning, noon, and night, that you can practice daily or as best fits in with your schedule.

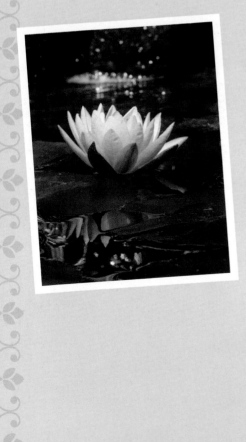

# 20-Minute Morning Practice

## WAKE UP AND GLOW!

Although waking up 20 minutes earlier may not initially appeal to you, I believe that once you have tasted this mood-lifting, endorphin-producing, and body-energizing practice you will bound out of bed before you can hit snooze. To start the day with intention and attention can ground and inspire you for hours, and even help you to sleep more soundly at night.

You can choose an intention by referring to one of the sections in Part 3 to inspire you (such as Confidence), or simply choose something that comes to mind. For example, it could be: "Today I will practice kindness and hold that as the center point for the day. I will be kind and gentle with myself, my family, and my friends, and kind to the Earth and all I come into contact with." Once you have articulated an intention for yourself or chosen one from Part 3, sit quietly and "breathe in" the intention until you feel connected and aligned to the essence of it. Come back to it periodically throughout the day. This practice can be very powerful, and it creates a positive and centered tone for your day.

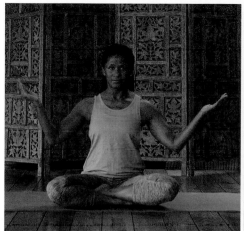 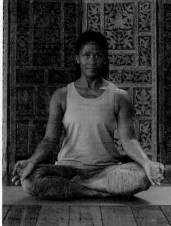 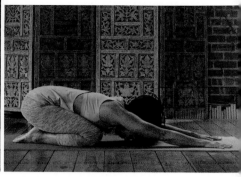

**1** Sit comfortably on the floor or in a chair. Rest your hands on your thighs or bring your arms into the Mudra for Receiving Energy by bending your elbows and holding your arms out from your body with the palms facing up. Set an intention for the day (see box, opposite). Take 10 *Ujjayi* breaths (page 28)—inhale through your nose while lightly constricting your throat so that your breath makes a "whoosh" sound. Exhale in the same manner, listening for that sound. On each inhale, pull your intention into your body and imagine it infusing every cell. On the exhales, soften into allowing the energy into your whole being.

**2** Skull Shining Breath with bandhas (page 119) for 3 rounds.

**3** Come into Child's Pose (page 12) with your big toes together and your knees apart, arms outstretched, for 5 breaths.

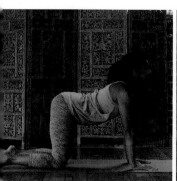 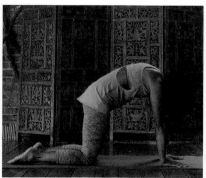 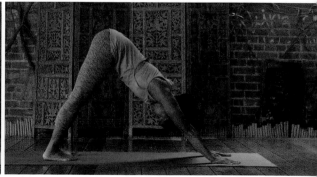

**4** On an inhale, move into Cat Cow Pose (pages 40–41) for 5 rounds. Inhale as you gently arch your back, opening your chest, and exhale as you pull the navel to the spine, making a dome with your back.

**5** From a flat back position, lift into Downward Dog (page 11). Root down into your feet, keeping your hips lifting and your heels descending. Spread the fingers wide and press the entire palm into the floor. Hold for 5 breaths.

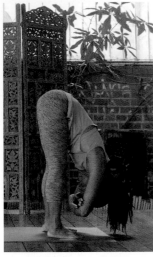
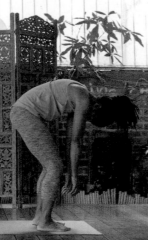
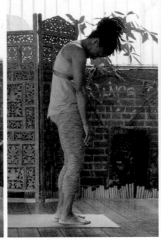
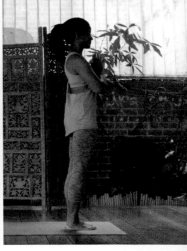

**6** Walk your hands to your feet, bending your knees as needed, coming into Standing Forward Fold (page 11), clasping your elbows for 3–5 breaths.

**7** Bend your knees, release your arms, and roll up to stand in *Tadasana* (page 9). Bring your hands to prayer position over the heart center (*Anjali Mudra*) for 2–3 breaths.

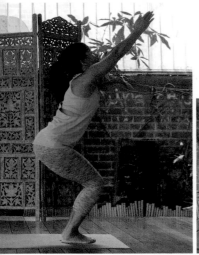
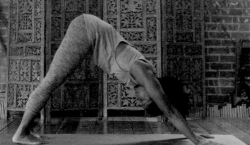
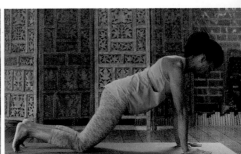

**10** Inhale as you lift your arms overhead and exhale as you bend at the hips, knees, and ankles, lowering your rear while stretching the torso upward into Chair Pose (pages 75–76). Keep your arms active and in line with your ears. Hold for 1–3 breaths.

**11** Step into Downward Dog (page 11) for one breath and then either roll forward to Plank Pose (pages 101–102) and lower to the floor slowly, or lower knees first, then chest, then chin.

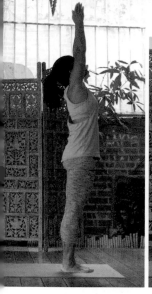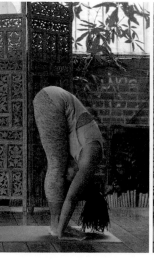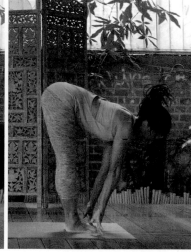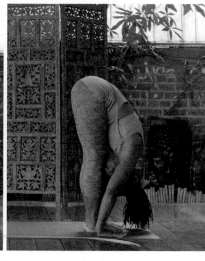

**8** On an inhale, sweep your arms overhead so the palms touch and, as you exhale, fold at the hips, hands to the floor, in a Standing Forward Fold.

**9** Inhale and lift your chest up, lengthening your spine into a Standing Half Forward Fold. Your arms are straight, and your hands are either touching the floor or on your shins. Exhale and fold forward again.

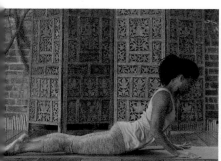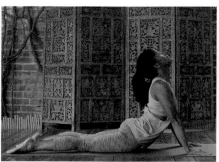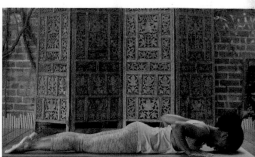

**12** Make sure your hands are right beneath your shoulders, pointing forward, and your elbows are bent backward. Root into your hips and pelvis, and inhale as you rise up into Cobra Pose (pages 43–44). Take 3 rounds, lifting on the inhale each time, pressing your legs firmly into the floor, and rolling slowly down the front of your body.

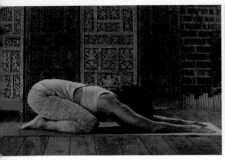

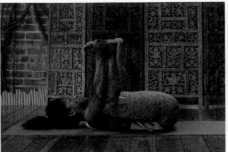

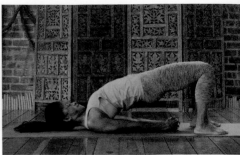

**13** Stretch back to Child's Pose for 2–3 breaths.

**14** Come onto your back for Happy Baby Pose. Lift the legs into the air, and bending at the knees, reach for your feet, ankles, or back of the knees. Breathe and relax for 3–5 breaths.

**15** Place your feet on the floor hip-width apart and parallel, and lift your hips into Bridge Pose (page 60). Interlace your hands underneath you and straighten your arms for 3–5 breaths. Slowly lower down from upper back to lower back, with your lower back coming into contact with the floor last.

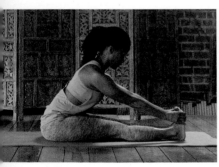

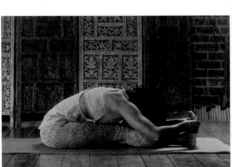

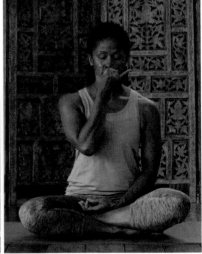

**18** Next come to a seated forward fold, Intense Stretch of the West (pages 64–65), for 3–5 breaths.

**19** Sit cross-legged in *Sukhasana* or *Siddhasana* (page 10), or choose another comfortable seated pose, and practice 9 rounds of Sun Breath (page 110).

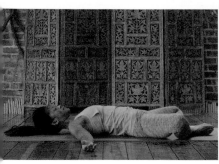
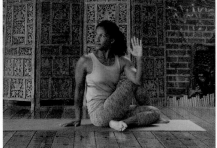
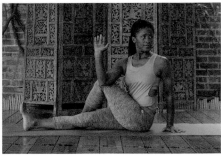

**16** Let your feet come together and your knees fall open to the floor, coming into Reclining Butterfly (pages 55–56) with just a low support for your head if necessary. Stay for a few breaths and then hug your knees into your chest.

**17** Sit up for a seated twist (*Matsyendrasana*) on both sides. Start with your legs out in front of you in *Dandasana* (page 9). Bend your left leg along the floor and place your left foot near to your right hip. Cross your right leg over your left with the knee bent and the foot on the floor near your left hip. Place your right hand behind your back on the floor, extend your left arm up, bend the elbow, and hook the elbow

outside your right knee. Gaze over your right shoulder, keeping your spine lifted. You could take the variation of Half Lord of the Fishes (page 64) by keeping your first leg straight out in front of you with the foot flexed, instead of bending it along the floor. Hold for 3–5 breaths before switching sides.

**20** Lie down in *Savasana* (page 13) for a few minutes. Alternatively, stay in seated meditation with Break of Day (*Ushas Mudra*, page 139). Enjoy a few moments of alert relaxation before heading into the rest of your day.

Have a glowing day!

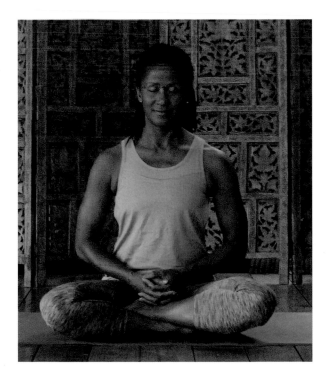

# Noon Sequence

## RESET AND REVIVE

This midday sequence can be done at any middle point or break time that works for you. If you are going to practice near lunchtime, practice first and eat after! Make sure you are hydrated and, if possible, change into comfortable clothes.

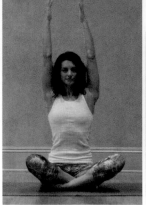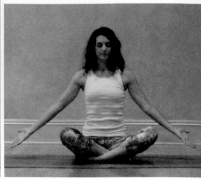

**1** Sit comfortably in *Sukhasana* (page 10) and lift your arms overhead. Inhale 3 sniffs or short breaths and exhale one longer, forceful breath through the nose. This is a rapid *Dirga* Breath (page 87). Practice 5 rounds, and on the last round exhale through the mouth and bring your arms down.

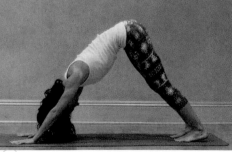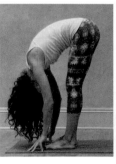

**High Plank into Cobra**

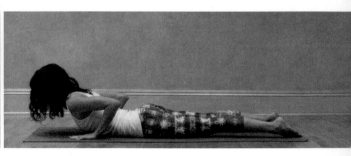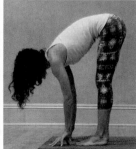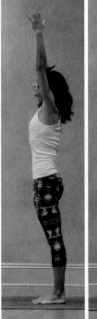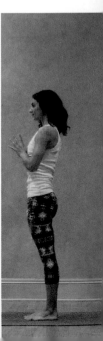

**Downward Dog into Standing Half Forward Fold and Standing Forward Fold, then back to *Tadasana***

**2** Come to standing and do 5–10 rounds of Sun Salutations A (pages 18–19). Choose whether to go from Half Standing Forward Fold to High Plank and Cobra before Downward Dog, or Low Plank and Upward Facing Dog.

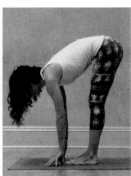

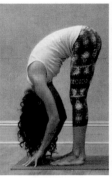

***Tadasana* into Standing Forward Fold, then Half Standing Forward Fold**

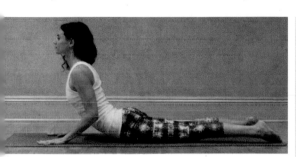

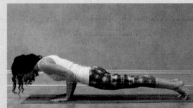

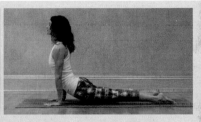

**Alternative: Low Plank into Upward Facing Dog**

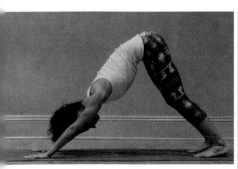

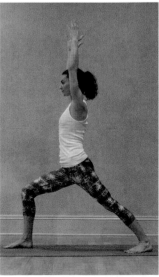

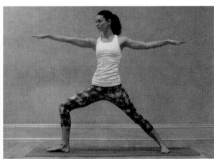

**3** Go into Downward Dog and step your right leg forward into Warrior I (pages 96–97). Take 3–5 breaths here with the legs strong and grounded and the arms lifting and energized. Step back to Downward Dog and repeat on the other side.

**4** From Downward Dog, step your right leg forward into Warrior II (page 98). Relax the shoulders, extend from heart to fingertips, and set your focus point (*drishti*) over the middle finger of your right hand. Take 3–5 breaths, step back to Downward Dog, and switch sides.

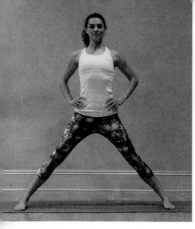
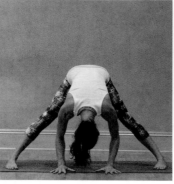
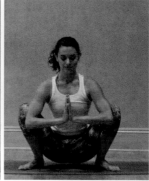
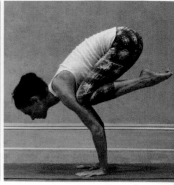

**5** From Warrior II on the left side, straighten your left leg and turn both feet so that they are parallel with each other. Place the hands on the hips and fold forward into Wide-legged Forward Fold (pages 58–59) for 5 breaths.

**6** Heel-toe your feet in from here and either squat into Garland Pose (page 48, with or without the mudra) or bend your elbows, lift your rear, and come into Crow Pose (pages 151–52). In either case, stay for as many breaths as is comfortable.

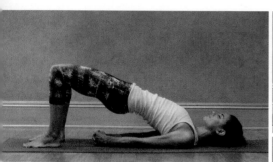
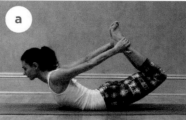
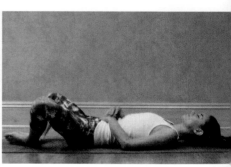

**9** If you are in tabletop position, lift into Downward Dog. Then walk your feet forward and lie down on your back. Place your feet under your knees, arms by your sides. Lift into Bridge Pose (page 60). Stay for 3–5 breaths and release.

**10** If you feel inspired, take a deep backbend with either Bow Pose (page 114) (**a**) or Wheel Pose (pages 126–27) (**b**). Hold for as long as you are comfortable and can breathe calmly.

**11** Release onto your back into Reclining Butterfly (pages 55–56), unsupported if possible.

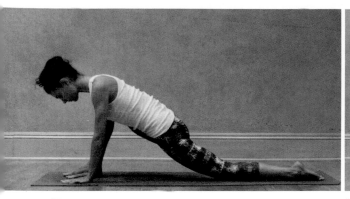

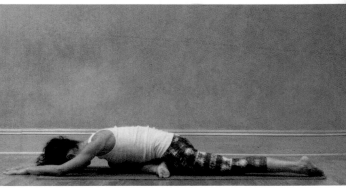

**7** Come out of the pose and into Low Lunge (pages 66–67) by stretching your left leg back and dropping the knee to the floor while placing your right foot under your bent right knee. Take 5 breaths here, then step back into Downward Dog or tabletop position and switch sides.

**8** From Downward Dog or tabletop position, bring your right leg forward for One-legged King Pigeon Pose (page 69). Hold for 3–5 breaths, then step back to Downward Dog or tabletop position and switch sides.

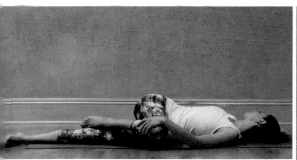

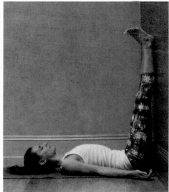

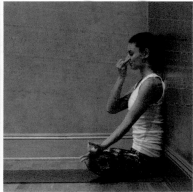

**12** Draw your knees into your chest and direct them toward the floor on one side, arms out straight from your shoulders, with your head turned the opposite way, for 3–5 breaths. Repeat on the other side. Alternatively, hug the right knee in and leave the left leg straight. Bring the knee across the leg toward the floor. Leave your right arm out straight and turn your head to the right. Hold for 3–5 breaths and repeat on the other side.

**13** Rest in either *Savasana* (page 13) or Legs up the Wall (page 30).

**14** If you prefer, come straight to a cross-legged position (*Sukhasana* or *Siddhasana*, page 10) for a seated meditation. Bring the thumbs, ring fingers, and pinky fingers together, and extend the index and middle fingers for *Prana Mudra* (page 110).

**15** Finish with Alternate Nostril Breathing (page 89) for 5–10 rounds, or longer if you like.

As you head into the rest of your day, acknowledge your efforts on behalf of yourself and all those you come into contact with. As you practice health and wellbeing, you bring light to the world and set an inspiring example for others.

# Nighttime Sequence

## EASE ON DOWN

This sequence is perfect for draining tension from the body and mind and preparing for a good night's sleep. It can be done any time in the evening, including right before bed. The spirit of the practice is to let go of the unfinished business of the day, release any grievances, and touch upon gratitude and contentment. Wear comfortable clothes and practice in a dim light (candles!) if possible.

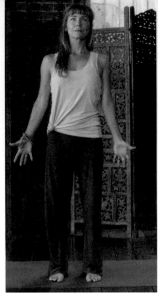

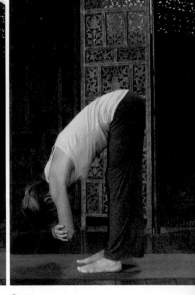

**1** Stand in *Tadasana* (page 9) with eyes open or closed. Imagine that you are standing in soft rain, being washed clean of any physical or mental stress that may have accumulated like dirt. Soften your shoulders and your face and take 5 slow breaths.

**2** Sweep your arms overhead as you inhale, and exhale into Standing Forward Fold (page 11). Clasp the elbows, relax the belly, and feel your head get heavy as gravity helps you to lengthen your neck. Imagine that soft rain on your lower back. Take 5 slow breaths.

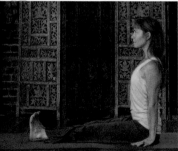
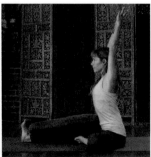
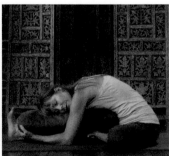
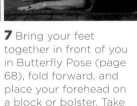

**6** Release your arms and come to sitting with both legs straight out in front of you in *Dandasana* (page 9). Draw your left leg back by the inner knee and bring the left foot to the inner right thigh. If you have a bolster or blankets, place them along your right leg. On an inhale, lift your arms overhead. As you exhale, twist your torso slightly to the right and extend down onto your leg or your support in Head to Knee Pose (pages 91–92). Turn your head to the side if you are supported, and take 5 breaths. Lift up slowly with your hands on the floor. Switch sides.

**7** Bring your feet together in front of you in Butterfly Pose (page 68), fold forward, and place your forehead on a block or bolster. Take 5 slow breaths.

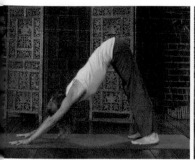

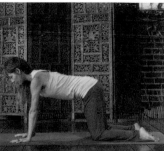

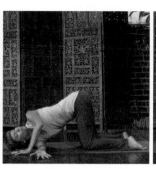

**3** Step into Downward Dog (page 11) and hold for 5 slow breaths.

**4** Bring your knees down into tabletop position and slide your right arm under your left arm for Revolved Child's Pose (page 42). Your left hand is right under your left elbow, and you are resting on the upper back right side of your head. Take 3–5 breaths here and repeat on the other side.

**5** Come back to tabletop position. Bring your big toes together and knees apart for Child's Pose (page 12). Then interlace your fingers behind you and lift the hands toward your shoulder blades and the sky. Take 3–5 breaths here with your chin tucked in.

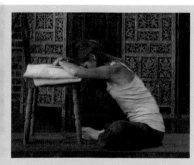

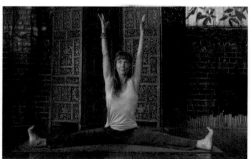

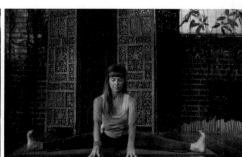

**7 alternative** Bring your feet together in front of you in Butterfly Pose (page 68), fold forward, and place your forehead on a folded blanket on a chair. Rest your forearms on the blanket. Take 5 slow breaths.

**8** Stretch your legs out to the sides in Straddle Stretch (*Uppavista Konasana*) and lift your arms overhead, lengthening your spine. Press your legs down and, as you exhale, bring your hands to the floor (**above right**). Alternatively, you could use a bolster propped on a block and lower your torso onto your support (**right**). Either turn your head to the side or place your forehead on your forearms. Take 5 breaths.

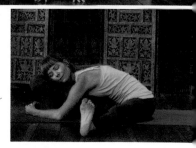

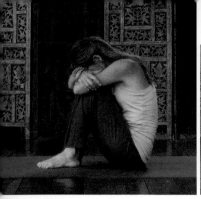

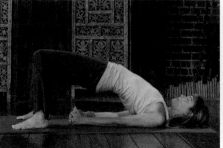

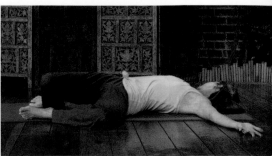

**9** Bend your legs by lifting from the backs of the knees and bring your feet to the floor, knees together. Cross your forearms and place them on your knees, and rest your head on your arms for Sage Pose. Relax face and eyes, imagine your mind softening and melting, and breathe. When you feel ready, lift your head and roll onto your back slowly, using your core muscles to ease your way down.

**10** Once you are on the floor with your feet under your knees, press your arms into the ground and lift your hips into Bridge Pose (page 60). Take 5 breaths as you open your heart in appreciation for the day and honor yourself and all your efforts, so finishing the day with compassion for yourself and an open heart.

**11** Lower down to the ground, leave the feet as they are, and drop both knees to the left. Roll your head to the right, stretching out your arms. Make sure to keep the space between your feet for this supine twist. Take 3–5 easy breaths here and repeat on the other side.

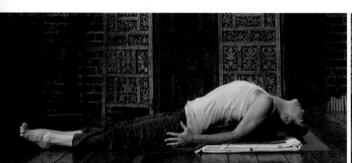

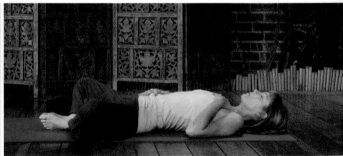

**13** From your position lying on your back, come into Fish Pose (*Matsyasana*) by pressing into your forearms and lifting your chest, allowing your head to move backward until the crown comes onto the floor. Keep the legs strong and engaged. If this is uncomfortable, try Supported Fish (page 36). After 3–5 breaths, relax your whole body onto the floor.

**14** Bring the feet together into Reclining Butterfly Pose (pages 55–56), unsupported. Place one hand on the heart and one hand on the belly. Inhale for 4 counts and exhale for 7 counts. If this is difficult, inhale for 2 counts and exhale for 5 counts. Repeat this cycle 5–10 times or for as long as you like. Place support under your knees if necessary, or stretch the legs out if you prefer.

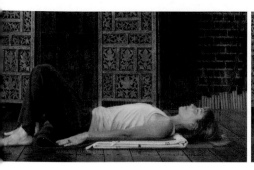
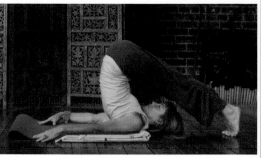
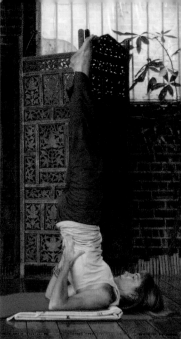

**12** Come into Shoulder Stand via the Plow (pages 35–36) if you want to. If not, you can skip ahead to Reclining Butterfly Pose. Once in Shoulder Stand, try to keep your elbows in line with your shoulders and your abdomen slightly engaged. Lift your chest toward your chin and press with medium pressure into the back of your head. Relax your face and throat and breathe naturally for 1–3 minutes. To come out, bend your knees and roll slowly from the top of your spine through to your lower spine to the floor.

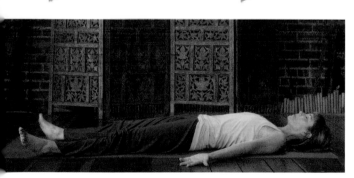

**15** Finish in *Savasana* (page 13), either flat or with your legs elevated with a bolster or blankets under the back of the knees. Alternatively, lie on your belly in Crocodile Pose (page 57), with your heels in and toes out. In Crocodile Pose, you can also place blankets or a bolster under your pelvis and hips for an extra yummy low-back release and a boost to your digestive system. Cross your arms and bow your head onto the arms.

As you rest in your final pose, make peace with the day. Remember that as you head toward slumber it is a time to regenerate and refresh. The most productive and healthful thing you can do is give yourself permission to press "pause." If you find that your mind is active, direct your thoughts to those that are comforting or revisit a few particularly pleasant moments in your day. Direct your attention away from things that stimulate or upset you, and don't try to finish or resolve anything at this time. Let your breath soothe you like a lullaby that was written just for you.

# Resources

There are many glorious and informative books and articles that I feel have found their way, directly or indirectly, into this book. My teaching and my journey have been shaped and touched by them. It could actually be an endless list of inspiration and information. However, I will offer you the most direct sources that actually made their way either into the pages or into the spirit of the book.

## Books

*Pocketful of Miracles* by Joan Borysenko (Warner Books, 1994)

*Mudras: Yoga in Your Hands* by Gertrud Hirschi (Red Wheel/Weiser, 2016)

*Light on Yoga* by B. K. S. Iyengar (Schocken Books, 1979)

*Yoga: The Path to Holistic Health* by B. K. S. Iyengar (Dorling Kindersley, 2014)

*Healing Mudras: Yoga for Your Hands* by Sabrina Mesko (The Ballantine Publishing Group, 2000)

*The Anatomy of the Spirit* by Caroline Myss (Three Rivers Press, 1996)

*The Yoga Sutras of Patanjali* by Sri Swami Satchidananda (Integral Yoga Publications, 1999)

*The Book of Chakras* by Ambika Wauters (Quarto Publishing, 2002)

*Yoga Beyond Belief* by Ganga White (North Atlantic Books, 2007)

## Book and CD sets

*The 7 Secrets of Sound Healing* by Jonathan Goldman (Hay House, 2008)

*The Divine Name: The Sound that Can Change the World* by Jonathan Goldman (Hay House, 2010)

*Healing Sounds: The Power of Harmonics* by Jonathan Goldman (Healing Arts Press, 2002)

*Shifting Frequencies: Sounds for Vibratory Activation* by Jonathan Goldman (Light Technology Publications, 1998)

*Tantra of Sound* by Jonathan Goldman and Andi Goldman (Hampton Road Publications, 2005)

*The Lost Chord* (Spirit Music, 2000) (CD only)

## Websites and articles

www.quizlet.com/24507436/yoga-pose-english-sanskrit-flash-cards
A guide to the Sanskrit names for yoga poses and terms.

www.smm.org/heart/lessons/lesson2.htm
Learn more about the heart and discover your cardiac output.

www.yogapedia.com/definition/6874/vajrapradama-mudra
Advice on the Vajrapradama Mudra.

www.jivamuktiyoga.com/focus/lokah-samastah-sukhino-bhavantu
Translation of the chant on page 123 by Sharon Gannon.

www.balayoga.com/om-lokah-samastah-sukhino-bhavantu
Further information on the chant on page 123.

www.mayoclinic.org/diseases-conditions/tension-headache/basics/causes/con-20014295
Causes of tension headaches.

www.yogajournal.com/slideshow/tap-power-tantra-yoga-sequence-confidence
"Tap the Power of Tantra: A Sequence for Self-Trust" by Jessie Lucier.

www.yogajournal.com/uncategorized/yoga-help-manage-ocd
"Yoga Could Help Manage OCD" by *Yoga Journal* editor.

www.yogamag.net/archives/1982/emay82/prana582.shtml
"Prana: The Universal Life Force" by Swami Satyananda Saraswati (*YOGA* magazine, 1982).

www.authenticityassociates.com/emotions-are-energy
"Emotions Are Energy" by Dr. Kim Ward and Dr. Hilary Stokes.

# Index

# Acknowledgments

It truly does take a village. When our child came out of my body, I was surrounded by loved ones and professionals. From inception through pregnancy, there was excitement, support, hand-holding, soothing, joy, and a dose of fear! This book was the same. Somehow acknowledging those who make up my village is a bit more daunting than writing the book! How far to go back? How far to expand my arms in embrace? It's entirely possible that I do not get this right, but perfection is not the goal, or shouldn't be; rather, the best of intentions and authentic deep appreciation are the fuel to find the direction for honoring those that have held my hand as this book was born.

Let me start by bowing deeply to the tradition of yoga itself, which was born so long ago, and all the gurus, teachers, and guides that protected, shared, and continue with the practice so that it is more alive and vibrant today than ever. From here, let me add my personal gurus and teachers who inspired, instructed, encouraged, and led by example so that I was moved to follow. They are, in order of appearance in my life: David and Sharon Gannon, Ganga White and Tracey Rich, Frank White, Steve Walter, Paul Cabanis, Ana Forrest, and Marla Apt. Many more spoke to me from the pages of books and through the airwaves, but these teachers I had the good fortune to experience firsthand. Then I would like to acknowledge and honor the teachers at Liberation Yoga who inspire me daily with their dedication, expertise, passion, and generosity of spirit.

With deep appreciation, I thank CICO Books, beginning with Kristine Pidkameny, commissioning editor. Through divine inspiration Kristine reached out to me and, along with the always lovely Cindy Richards, offered me this golden opportunity. Kristine and I shared heartfelt conversations about yoga and the essence of the book, and her touch is felt throughout. I thank Cindy for her foolproof eye for truth and beauty, which shaped and guided this process every step of the way. Adding into the delicious mix that is CICO is Carmel Edmonds. I am in awe of her editorial talents that range from minute details to the grandest concepts, and her cheery and gentle demeanor, which kept my spirits high as she whittled down my words so deftly. Thank you to Marion Paull, whose sharp eye and keen knowledge of yoga caught mistakes, posed excellent questions, and made sure the book didn't turn out like a game of Twister! Geoff Borin, Sally Powell, and Kerry Lewis, I applaud you vigorously for sorting through the plethora of poses and words and making such beautiful sense of it all!

A huge bouquet of appreciation goes to my agent, Kari Stuart and her assistant, Patrick Morley, at ICM, who have made this process sweeter and made it possible for me to create the time to write.

I must extend a huge loving hug to Erika Flores (photographer extraordinaire), who waded through thousands of Sanskrit names, hiked to the top of a mountain and into the ocean with me, and always smiled and brought so much love to the process. I express much gratitude to the models, who were all Liberation teachers and the dearest of people: Shanna Gilfix, Pat Sperry, Joella Enderes, Bahni Turpin, and Johnny Asuncion.

Special thanks to dear ones: Caleb, Frank, June, Pamela, Gabe, Pagan, Will, Quinn, Tom, and Nicole, who celebrate and support me. With deep love and endless gratitude for always making me feel invincible, I honor my sister, Brittany, brother, Drew, and my stepfather, Dave. Lastly I send love to dog heaven and my writing partner, Mattie, who will not see the publication of the book, but was with me every day of the process.